CW01512920

About the author

Jules Von Hep is a celebrated beauty expert, body confidence advocate, and co-founder of Isle of Paradise (departing in February 2025). Known for his vibrant energy and unapologetic authenticity, Jules began as a celebrity spray tanner, working backstage at fashion weeks and with A-list stars. He quickly became known not just for his golden glow techniques, but for his infectious message of self-love. A fierce champion of body confidence, Jules uses his platforms to empower others, reminding everyone that confidence is a ritual – one that begins from within. Jules has been interviewed many times, and has appeared in and/or written for *Vogue, Harper's Bazaar, The Times, Telegraph, HELLO!, Red, Grazia* and the *Evening Standard*.

JULES VON HEP

The

Confidence

Ritual

Give Yourself a Glow up From the Inside Out

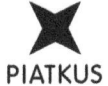

PIATKUS

PIATKUS
First published in Great Britain in 2025 by Piatkus
1 3 5 7 9 10 8 6 4 2

A CIP catalogue record for this book
is available from the British Library.

ISBN: 978-0-34944-389-8

Typeset in Bembo by Hewer Text UK Ltd, Edinburgh
Printed and bound in Great Britain by Clays Ltd, Elcograf S.p.A.

Papers used by Piatkus are from well-managed forests
and other responsible sources.

Piatkus
An imprint of
Little, Brown Book Group
Carmelite House
50 Victoria Embankment
London EC4Y 0DZ

The authorised representative
in the EEA is
Hachette Ireland
8 Castlecourt Centre, Dublin 15,
D15 XTP3, Ireland
(email: info@hbgi.ie)

An Hachette UK Company
www.hachette.co.uk

www.littlebrown.co.uk

I dedicate my ritual to you. Past, present, future – every version, every era, every layer of wonderful you. Where you are, right now, today, this very moment is exactly where you are supposed to be. Whatever your unique version of rising phoenix might look like, allow yourself to conjure it up as you digest these pages. Something has brought this ritual into your life – my advice is 'Lean in and roll with it, babes!'

Contents

Introduction

'You must think well of yourself. You must see yourself
as worth celebrating, worth loving, worth having.'
Angelina Talpa, author & lifestyle coach

Throughout the course of your life, the most important conversations you'll ever have are the ones you will have with yourself. The tone of that inner dialogue – the very words you use – is more important than you may realise. For years now, for decades, too many of us have overlooked the severity of self-deprecating dialogue and the damage that can do to our self-belief and self-respect. Too often – until it's pointed out by someone else – the way we talk to and about ourselves, internally and externally, can keep us in a place of low-vibe dullness. We all deserve to be spoken to with kindness, and this starts with every one of us being our own advocate and cheerleader.

How can we glow when our inner chat is mean or dull? The dark mist of horrid inner talk sits low in our hearts, meaning we're unable to see our value and worth clearly.

When our inner dialogue is nothing but negative, the heavy impact on our day-to-day life is huge. From the start of each day, from the very moment we open our eyes, our brain gets flooded with a swirling fog of low vibrations and low moods.

I understand how easy it is to get trapped in this horrible hurricane. For years I was stuck in a cycle of thinking the worst, saying the worst, and believing the worst about myself. I was my biggest critic when I should have been my loudest champion. Today, I stand corrected and my world has shifted skywards towards the sun, my inner vibrations raised through the roof. I went from hating every inch of who I was to standing proud of everything I have achieved, confident in the skin I'm in – my wobbles and all!

And I want to share how I changed my life – and destiny – with you. Throughout my career, from working backstage at fashion shows and on film sets as a celebrity spray tanner to becoming a global beauty brand founder, of Isle of Paradise, I have gathered invaluable tools, tips and methods to boost my self-belief. And now I'm ready to teach them all to you. Over the following pages I hope you will allow me to be your guide to inner and outer confidence, and to help you become the person you always wanted to be; the you that has always been there, just hidden behind negativity and doubt.

Relearning how you think and talk about yourself won't be easy at times, believe me. That negative inner voice can be so persuasive – dictating or limiting us in every way, from the goals we set ourselves, to the circles we move in, even to the job and partner we choose. If the chips are down, it can feel like nothing really flows as it's supposed to. Even in a place of perceived happiness we can be unhappy. Life might look to the outside world as if everything is flowing in abundance: we have our health, we're in our dream job, we might even have the body of our dreams … On paper it may seem like we've got everything we could ever have wished for. We might have all the material objects our heart desires (the house, the car, the family, the wardrobe), but there's still something missing. We know, deep down, that we're not happy.

BEEN THERE, DONE THAT

Only a few years ago, I can remember emitting a heavy sigh when I looked at myself in the mirror every morning. Like clockwork: the sun comes up, a sigh comes out, setting my low mood and low expectations for the day. Yes, every morning I started my day with a nothingness tone, with an attitude that felt tight and desolate instead of being filled with abundance and joy. Perhaps you can relate? Or maybe you feel on edge or filled with anxiety, worried that something isn't clicking into place or is harder than it should be – you haven't got the promotion you deserve, or met the love of your life, when all your friends are climbing the career ladder and coupled up, perhaps? Do you ask yourself, 'How come everyone else has everything I want, but I don't have it?' Maybe you feel a different negative emotion as you start each day.

Up until ten years ago, the way I spoke to myself wasn't how I'd speak to my friends, family or clients – or even to strangers. Rather than walk into a room knowing I'd light it up, I just coasted through my day, keeping my head down, a life lived on autopilot. I willingly took a back seat in my own existence, believing I couldn't achieve greatness or get what I desired. I told myself my body was the problem. I repeatedly focused on everything in my life that I deemed wrong, rather than championing what I felt was right. I cheered on everyone else – but never cheered on myself.

I learned to loathe my appearance and personality and spent too many years in both childhood and adulthood hating how I looked, how I acted . . . hating everything about myself. I believed that what I saw in advertising campaigns, magazine articles and social media was the truth: that my worth was solely a reflection of the number on the weighing scales or in the size label in my clothes. I placed a lot of my worth on materialism and aesthetics. Sure, I used all the glow-giving make-up products ever invented, but my inner dullness never brightened. I had no confidence; I had no real glow.

And then out of the darkness, after twenty years' hating who I was, a few simultaneous 'flash bulb' moments in my personal and professional life led me to an inner awakening. The light finally came to me from within. I began to carve out my own personal ritual, the very ritual that lies within this book. The ritual I am going to teach YOU. Small changes that are simple to make and that over time can change the course of your life immeasurably. I decided I wasn't going to be that negative person any more. I wanted to feel alive. Are you the same? Are you with me?

Firstly, good – you're asking yourself questions. Secondly, I'm glad you've picked up this book because it tells me you're prepared to make some changes to stop yourself feeling so low. I know right now that everything seems harder and darker than it should, but reading and doing the exercises laid out in *The Confidence Ritual* will boost your vibe. What do I mean by that? Well, the way I see it, your vibe is like your mood, but it's more constant: it's what you give out to the world for others to connect with. If you're feeling down and your overarching self-belief is minimal, that is what you'll portray to others as you make your way through life.

For years, I knew that I'd lost – or had never truly had – that spring in my step that others seemed to have so easily. Pessimism ruled my inner thought processes. I was consistently negative and my energy flowed downwards. I didn't even know the capabilities of my inner power, let alone how to step into it.

That is no way to live – not for me, and not for you. I knew I could be better, do better, live better. I knew a fire needed to be lit. I hope *The Confidence Ritual* can act as your fire as you allow me to be your teacher. Prepare to learn about yourself, and get ready to grow.

TASTE FOR LIFE

Whenever I'm hosting confidence workshops, I get people thinking about their futures by using the analogy of sushi rolls whizzing past customers in a Japanese restaurant. If you're not familiar with how a sushi belt works, fresh sushi is placed on different colour plates on a moving conveyor belt that passes diners. Each plate colour falls into a different price bracket and at the end, your total bill will get worked out depending on the number and colour of plates of raw fish and rice delights you have grabbed off the moving carousel. One by one the sushi rolls are put on the belt, shiny and new, on their variously priced plates. Whirring round and round, being scooped up by hungry people choosing the plates that look the most desirable. What am I drawn to? What seems appealing?

Now stick with me. If we don't implement change, or the work that is needed, our vibe isn't put into place and we become a bit like a California Roll. Yes, it's a classic sushi roll consisting of crab, avocado and cucumber covered with sushi rice and orange roe, but . . . They look good when they're first assembled – not the most exciting or tasty, but a safe choice – until they've been on the belt a bit too long, monotonously going round and round, becoming a little more colourless and unappetising with each lap. At that point your gut tells you to avoid that plate. Perhaps like an old California Roll, you're getting a bit stale around the edges. Perhaps you're not looking or feeling your best – tired, flat, not quite what you looked like when you first jumped on the belt – when, bang! The next thing you know, a Dragon Roll has been placed next to you. Now, Dragon Rolls are usually expensive sushi rolls, displayed on a golden plate. The Dragon Roll is open, crispy, fresh, exotic, enticing. Everyone is looking admiringly at the Dragon Roll.

So, yes, I'm likening low-vibe you to a bit of raw fish, but you get what I mean? What do you want to be: a tired California Roll . . . or a Dragon Roll? Until you realise you've been sat on the sushi belt, going round and round, getting slowly less appetising, and getting upstaged by better sushi, you might not even know there's a problem. But I'm here to help: do you want to be placed in the reduced sushi section, or is it time to step into your Dragon Roll era?

Now, I don't know you and I'm unsure of where you're at right now, whether you're in search of something to enrich your life, or looking for that thing that makes you glow, or perhaps searching for a whole new and different version of you. Maybe it's simpler than that – you could just do with a boost? I get it! And I am here for all of it, for all of you, and whatever vibe lift you need right now. By the end of the book, my goal is for you to be able to talk to yourself in the same way I am going to talk to you throughout its pages: with love, with kindness, with acceptance and with a hell yeah! You got this, babes.

LET THE SUN SHINE IN

When I'm giving interviews, or when I'm being announced on stage as a global beauty brand founder or a well-being keynote speaker, I'm regularly referred to as *human sunshine*. The old me can't believe that I now host confidence workshops around the world, teaching individuals the art of glowing at their truest potential. I started from a place where I hated every single aspect of who I was, picking myself apart every minute of every day, and yet now I stand in front of crowds teaching them the skills to becoming more confident. I own my wobbles when I look in the mirror and I've taught myself to not only accept it, but to love it. My wobbles are part of what makes me who I am. Whether it's physical or mental, we all wobble in some way.

Having worked in the beauty industry for nearly two decades, with a career predominantly centred on getting people ready for big moments – be it Hollywood actresses on the red carpet, models for magazine cover shoots or mothers of the bride – I've spent hour upon hour helping people to look their best. I'm paid to get other people ready; this is my bread and butter. When my now husband proposed, and I – as do many brides – entered the state of 'big event preparation perfection' panic, I properly understood how these huge eyes-on-you moments are so important ... but it also renewed my belief that how you feel inside is more important (and more beautifying) than how you look on the outside.

Maybe we're too focused on the exterior these days. When I'm getting people ready for their big moments, they chat away about the same, common obsessions. It's all about outfits, skin texture, body shape and weight ... all totally aesthetic goals. I rarely hear a goal that focuses on the inside – how come no one talks about our confidence as part of the getting-ready process? Rather than our confidence being a temporary knock-on effect resulting from a few beauty treatments, what if it was the main pillar of focus?

On the run-up to our wedding in 2022, I decided I wasn't going to diet for the big day. Having battled eating disorders and low self-esteem for many years, I knew that putting myself on a pre-wedding diet wasn't going to be a good choice for my mental health in the long run. Rather than my target being a smaller stomach, I was going to go on a self-love journey. My goal for my wedding day was to feel like the best version of me as I walked down the aisle. Instead of focusing the day on my outside, I focused my day on my inside. I chose *feeling* over aesthetic. It was the best decision I ever made, and I've stayed with that permanent glow up ever since!

WHAT IS A GLOW UP?

Whether you're working towards a specific date – maybe it's a wedding, a work promotion, or a family holiday, or you simply want to feel better in yourself moving forward – the ritual of your glow up shouldn't ever be viewed as something selfish or indulgent. It is all good . . . for you and those around you.

- A glow up can be a life's work: it becomes your ritual. Unlike a diet where we can reach a goal and stop, a glow up is the full 360 forever. Body confidence and self-worth is not the destination – it's a repeated process.
- A glow up isn't about simply buying a new beauty product or upping the number of squats you do in the gym. It's about doing deep-rooted inner work and stepping into your power.
- A glow up starts by recognising the person you are, and the person you want to become. It's the journey to finding a more confident you, and staying on the journey moving forward.
- A glow up mindset will teach you it is possible to gain inner and outer confidence and to make peace with your body.

DOES SELF-CARE COUNT?

Unfortunately, the world of marketing and social media has attempted to latch onto the concept of self-care in order to sell products and make money – not to help people do the deep work to get to a long-lasting healthier place. I urge you to look beyond that. You can perform self-care without buying products. Yes, a bath and a beauty evening *are* self-care – and I will really lean into the beautification process later in this book – but remember that there are so many other forms of self-care too. To me, self-care has profound healing abilities, for mind, body and soul. I urge you to really think about what could help your day-to-day life, rather than give you a quick fix (and a dent in your wallet).

Before I really learned about self-care, I felt lost. It felt like something was permanently missing from within. It was as if I was looking for something, but I didn't know what. The elevated joy self-care can bring, and the deeper connection with my inner thoughts, has enabled me to live life in a spiritually richer way. Self-care has hugely helped with my anxiety levels and my, at times, depressive nature. And whenever I perform acts of self-care I also find it extremely useful to categorise them, to monitor that I'm doing enough each week. It can be easy to fall off the wagon or neglect self-care and then, I find, it's harder to start performing acts of self-kindness again. We may even return to the state of unsettled surface-level vibrations we were experiencing previously.

SHINE AUTHENTICALLY

We've all heard the phrase 'fake it till you make it' and while I understand where this is coming from, especially in a work sense, sadly it doesn't apply to confidence. Being authentically you is a direct result of deep-rooted self-care. If we are insecure, or our ego sits at the surface of who we are – we lack authenticity. As you work through *The Confidence Ritual* hopefully you will begin to realise that your authentic, true self is worth so much more than being an imposter in your own existence, trust me . . . it doesn't suit you. You may even start to recognise a lack of authenticity elsewhere; it's easy to spot – the energy someone gives out feels off, it's as if there's a dullness in their presence. Being truly authentic will directly impact your confidence. Take it from me, honey, self-confidence is the best outfit you can rock because when you master the art of inner confidence, no one can copy it. There's no dupe of authentically you so dig deep and shine bright!

HOW THIS BOOK WORKS

I've spent the past eight years reprogramming my entire life with ideas that I have now turned into *The Confidence Ritual*. It's changed who I am, how I operate, why I wake up in the morning, and what I leave my house for. Now, I'm going to teach it to you.

In Part One, I'll share the defining moments, lessons and beliefs from my life that have helped me carve out a new path and new ideas – my theory, if you will. Using personal anecdotes and lessons learned, we'll go through the road map of how you're feeling now, and why. I'll share the tools and tips I've used and taught to get people ready to revolutionise their well-being and mindset.

Part Two is more practical. I will lead you day by day through the readjustments and reboots you can implement in your life to really get up and glow. I have compiled a daily and weekly checklist – Ritual Bingo – which, I hope, will keep you on the track that leads to boosting your confidence, with lots of practical exercises along the way. I suggest that you read each chapter in Part Two the night before the day that chapter focuses on. For example, read the Sunday section on a Saturday evening. If you can, read the chapter again (or at least the easy-to-digest recap which I've called Thoughts of the Day) on the day it's intended, too. If you work shifts, or you work outside of the Monday-to-Friday routine, I recommend starting with Sunday (even if your Sunday is actually Tuesday!), and taking it from there. Use the guide in a way that best suits your week. Each day is designed to be read more than once until it starts to stick. You might not pick it all up in one go, and that's OK. Keep coming back for a memory refresh. This is a big lifestyle change, and it takes commitment and time.

All this change might feel gritty and uncomfortable at first, but I've lived through it, and I know you can too. The phoenix is not just a mythological creature, it's an energy; and I know you can truly embody the vibrations of a phoenix and rise out of the ashes!

THE CONFIDENCE RITUAL . . .

- Promises to bring you inner light, happiness and enriched fulfilment.
- Takes your focus away from your – or anybody else's – body shape, career status, or anything remotely revolving around hierarchy.
- Frees you from diet culture and materialism.
- Teaches you to speak to yourself with *respect*, to choose clothes that make you *feel good*, and be with people who *spark joy*.
- Encourages you to live a life where you make decisions based on whether or not they will improve the quality and energy of your entire life.

It's worth it. If you're not feeling your best right now, take it from me:

You have the power to walk into a room and light it up.
You have the power to not second-guess yourself.
You have the power to stop hating your body.
You have the power to believe in your abilities.

As we work through the book together, try not to expect results overnight. The quicker the win, the quicker the fall. As we reprogramme your day from routine to ritual, it can take time for the process to really kick in. Routine is not ritual. Routine is a set of repeated actions that become a habit. When you take an existing routine and add a sense of meaning, purpose, awareness and intent, it becomes a ritual. It's about bringing in the why. Consciously curating your routine, asking yourself why you're doing what you're doing and if it's bringing you true happiness and inner joy. This is how we slowly turn routine into ritual. Remember, patience is an asset. In today's world, where almost everything is available at the click of a button, confidence, unfortunately, isn't on next-day delivery. It requires work, but it will eventually become second nature. The tasks and changes I set you can be doubled up, done in tandem, or completed one after the other, and you'll learn to work smart. Before you know it, this place where you are now – just beginning or revisiting the ritual – will feel like a million moons ago.

The good news is that all the power I want to give you is already inside you. I've designed this book to help bring it out; to show you how to cultivate your inner fire, to rebirth your sparkling phoenix, to bring your strength and confidence out into the world. Once we realise that we are our own motivator, friend and inspiration, we will not only glow on the inside, but on the outside, too. And when you flow in that glowing state of self-assurance and self-confidence, the world will become your oyster, babes. Let's go!

Part One

The Road Map to Self-confidence

'It is not what happens to you, but how you react to it that matters.'
Epictetus, early Greek philosopher

When I was at my lowest, I couldn't see the wood for the trees. I felt like having inner confidence and vibrating on a high frequency were things destined for other people. I couldn't comprehend where to start or how to begin to make improvements. I knew there was masses of advice about self-love both online and in the workplace, but, from what I could see, there was very little education on the actual, daily steps needed to implement a self-confidence boosting self-care routine that worked. Well, no more! I am here to help.

DEMON DAYS

Imagine a life where you don't hate your body or wake up dreading another day flooded with insecurity and self-doubt. Picture this: the size of your waist doesn't matter, your thigh shape or gap is irrelevant. A life where, instead of constantly

punishing your body, you stop hating and start appreciating . . .
It *is* possible. And I'm going to get you there.

It's going to take some hard work. Every day we're fed thousands of images, many of them airbrushed, filtered, well lit,
distorted in some way or even 100 per cent false, made up by
someone at a computer with AI. We're shown pictures of
models or celebrities in campaigns selling us a version of a
fictional idealised life for us to aspire to, banishing our contentment and distorting the value we place on our own existence.
Aspiring to a world that doesn't even exist. Made to feel attain-
able, but completely unattainable. All to make money? Yep.

Without realising it, we can quickly fall into the repetitive
trap of feeling lesser, where every day we repeat what's wrong
with ourselves during the ever-flowing internal dialogue in
our brain. Constantly picking on faults, looking for change.
Rather than focusing on what we have, we focus on what we
don't have. Draining the feel-good tank and – more
importantly – our overall self-esteem.

I spent twenty years hating who I was, hating my body, focusing on how I looked in pictures, focusing on what I wasn't
achieving, and each time my mind went to these hateful places,
my self-esteem would plummet. I feel like I've been on every
single diet going: you name it, I've done it. This led to eating
disorders, anxiety, depression and feeling rock-bottom in myself.
I placed my entire worth on the size of my stomach and my love
handles. I based my worth in society on the shape of my body.

While on the outside I may have seemed relatively OK (I
paid my rent on time, had a good job, dated, socialised and
travelled), when I was alone with the mirror, I was unhappy with
who looked back at me. I believed something was wrong with
me. The inner dialogue I had with myself was troublesome.

At my lowest point I wrote a suicide note. I contemplated ending my life because I felt like I didn't deserve a place on this Earth. That level of lowness shaped my twenties. Partying hard to numb how I felt on the inside. Believing that this was it, this was how I was going to be for the rest of my life. When I started my career and moved to London, I experienced loneliness like nothing I'd known before. A huge and bustling city, full of millions of people, and I felt lonely. I'm sharing this because I want you to know that I understand and relate to how it feels to hate who you are on the inside and the outside. I've been there. I was there for twenty years. So much time wasted.

MY TURNAROUND

I've had an unusual career. Accidentally ending up as a celebrity spray tanner in my twenties – unsurprisingly a profession my schoolteachers failed to suggest to me – I've had experiences many wouldn't believe. The things I've seen, darling! I was trained in spray tanning by celebrity facialist and wellness guru Nichola Joss. Nichola taught me how to navigate and work with VIPs, how to command the energy within the beauty workspace and how to recognise that while the beauty industry weaves itself in and out of so many other industries where it's easy to get carried away (fashion, music, Hollywood …), the most important thing is staying true to who you are and keeping your feet firmly on the ground. I've worked on TV shows including *The X Factor*, *Strictly Come Dancing* and *The Crown*, plus endless glossy photoshoots … and all of those high-end fashion shows from New York to Milan, London to Paris. Celebrity clientele?! Babes, I've seen almost every celebrity naked. I became one of the, if not *the*, best spray tanners in the world, in and out of celebrity homes and quoted in all the bestselling magazines and newspapers. Having founded globally recognised self-tan brand Isle of Paradise, I'm the most successful spray tan artist in the world.

At one point in my career, I didn't dare leave the house without my passport and a tanning mousse and mitt. At any moment a celebrity agent might phone with a job in another country, and I'd have to drop everything there and then and go because 'no one else' would do! I once flew to Melbourne, Australia from London Heathrow (a twenty-six-hour flight) just to give someone a spray tan – I'm *that* good! Flying around the world to give people a glow up. I was – and still am – paid to look at naked bodies. Not many people can say that! I've worked with A-listers, Victoria's Secret models, politicians, DJs, pop stars – even princesses – but also accountants, teachers, nurses, marketing executives and clients having chemotherapy. You name it, I've tanned it.

Being exposed to such varying levels of social status, wealth, wellness, personality and – most of all – shape and size, helped to change my perspective on life and myself. Little shocks me now. I've seen it all – every type of perky or droopy body part, every dimple, endless scars, surprising body hairs, and my lord, every single bodily smell you could imagine. That's the beauty of spray tanning: you stop being weirded out by the human body, because frankly, *it's just a human body.* Whatever you think you have, I'll tell you now – someone has the same, if not a more extreme version.

All that endless nudity during photo shoots means I've experienced a secret only a handful of people in the world know: how to decipher what's real and what's airbrushed, and how to navigate life without falling into the trap of body hatred.

Prior to a spray tan, everything has to come off. Clothes, jewellery, make-up, deodorant – and if you don't want tan lines, underwear. I saw hundreds of people every single week, stripped down. Nothing to hide behind, no camouflage. Bare. When I put a hairnet on them and look into their eyes as we chat away, it feels like I can see into their soul. Some are kind and gentle, some funny; I can see the deep-rooted trauma or sadness, the ebb and flow of a someone's energy. All the light and dark inside a person becomes visually present, because there's nothing to hide behind. No visual distraction. That's the beauty of nudity.

Spray tanning saved me. It changed my perception of aesthetic and showed me true beauty. I learned that being beautiful isn't about the size of your stomach – it's goes much deeper than that.

So how much worth do you place on the size of your body, the shape of your nose, the thickness of your hair or the length of your legs, and whether you may or may not have cellulite? Concerns about my body size plagued me for years. I continually fell on and off the diet wagon, endlessly promising myself 'the diet starts tomorrow'. I reached my designated goal weight multiple times, only for it not to be good enough when I got there. I thought that reaching that certain number on a weighing machine would equal happiness and confidence, and that the universe would bring me everything I wanted because I'd starved myself. I was tired and hungry, but I was thin and surely that's all that mattered? Being thin. Because thin supposedly equalled being happy. It didn't.

My self-esteem was still in the gutter. I was living a life that felt unattainable, unhealthy and mentally exhausting. I realised that what was on the outside wasn't the issue, and that constantly trying to modify what was on the surface wasn't the answer. After seeing and spraying a sea of naked people's nipples and dimples – many of whom were unhappy with their appearance, however rich, or famous, or lusted after – I realised that everyone hates a part of their body.

I didn't want to be part of that negative noise any more.

I decided to find another way. I decided to say 'Yes!' to life. My body wasn't the problem: my viewpoint was. My mission was to stand tall, be confident and glow from the inside out. I needed to show myself respect and practise being my own best friend. Rather than living life constantly unhappy with my appearance I was going to truly step into my power. I was tired of hating how I looked, so I set out to teach myself how to make peace with my body and my appearance. A journey of self-discovery, rather than a diet. A journey built upon learnings, evidence and most of all: FEEL-GOOD VIBES. Restriction was out, self-love was in. I finally knew that . . .

- Confidence is a learned behaviour – it's more than a personality trait – it's a vibe!
- Being confident doesn't mean flashing a flat stomach or having a nice car parked in front of a big house. Confidence can't be bought.
- Confidence is about reaching a higher level of purpose.
- It's about leaving your house every day with authenticity, closing the front door behind you as you head into the world being sure of yourself without being arrogant.
- It's about knowing that who you are is good enough.
- Confidence is about healthy living, in both mind and body.
- Confidence and joy are interlinked – don't overlook that.

In this book there won't be any mention of calories, pounds, kilograms or dress sizes – this is deeper than metrics, babes! This is about stepping into your power. Stepping into *who you really are*. This is about glowing deeper and reaching a confidently clear lifestyle. Fear not, I won't be asking you to join a cult – I speak to you as a friend, who wants to make you feel better. It's as simple as that.

HOLDING ON AND LETTING GO

As we work through *The Confidence Ritual*, you may come to realise that you're holding on to moments or fragments from your past. Fragments that, instead of bringing you joy, bring you sadness. Perhaps this practice prevents you from truly stepping into your power?

We have all experienced comments that we hold on to. Some might just have been throwaway comments from a stranger, or from another child at school. Maybe an ex said something to you that you can't shake, or a family member had a certain phrase they used as you were growing up. These comments, over time, get pushed deeper and deeper into our core, eventually becoming part of who we are. Comments lodged in our inner psyche, knotted, forming part of our internal monologue and composition. And if we don't believe in our capabilities and magic, our self-esteem never really rises because every day we carry these negative things from the past.

Sometimes we don't realise where our self-esteem is at until we press pause. When self-esteem is low it affects our social life, our careers, our love life, our relationships with family and friends as well as the boundaries we may or may not have in place to protect our vulnerable side. Indeed, when our self-esteem is vibrating low, it affects multiple aspects of our existence and prevents us from becoming the best version of ourselves. We need to learn how to let go of the elements that hold us back. Remember that multiple factors such as environment, social media and past learned behaviour come into the equation, too.

We might not realise how other people already see us, how they *feel* the energy we give out. They may not be aware of our true inner power. What if we're already vibrating at a high frequency but we're just not tuned into it yet? Almost as if the final piece of the jigsaw is needed for us to work out how totally and utterly amazing we are?! The scenery doesn't need to change, but the viewpoint does. My life as a spray tanner and brand founder meant that I met hundreds, if not thousands, of people every single month, and now as a public speaker I'm meeting even more. People going about their lives who can't see or feel their true potential. People who I deem amazing, but can't see it in themselves at all.

There is no magic wand we can wave to bestow confidence on us, but we can conjure up confidence in ourselves with tricks or illusions, carving out a truly magical new version of us that we earn and that we deserve. As we work through *The Confidence Ritual* you may feel difficult moments from the past come to the surface. Please don't push them back down. Allow them to come up, and sit with them. I have cried multiple times writing this very book, so allow the feelings to surface. It's part of the process. Feel how the comments or moments affected you. As you do the work to raise your inner vibrations and boost your self-esteem, working through these moments will help you glow forward.

Self-love is true magic in helping to raise your inner frequency. If you want to journal out how you feel, I encourage you to do so. Why not pick up a notebook or journal now, and write down any standout moments that you feel have affected your confidence.

1

The Glow Up

I love – and live by – this quote from the sixth-century BCE Chinese philosopher Lao-Tzu:

'Watch your thoughts, they become words.
Watch your words, they become actions.
Watch your actions, they become habits.
Watch your habits, they become character.
Watch your character, it becomes your destiny.'

Bad habits form and happen to us all, vices come in all shapes and sizes and addictions can take our lives in a direction where they perhaps aren't meant to go. What if you're addicted to speaking to yourself badly? What if this negative self-chat is your vice? If you say mean things to yourself every day, and this has become your go-to thought process, then this is a habit: it's not reality. We're flooded with material to help us quit smoking or go sober, but what if you want to quit speaking to yourself badly?

This is where it stops! This is where an evolution takes place and you quit the negative inner dialogue.

The term *glow up* often refers to an aesthetic change on the outside, a rapid transformation, and – at times – a quick fix.

While there are elements of the shorter-term glow up that I relate to and practise myself, here and now we are referring to a ritualistic lifelong glow up.

Take make-up, for example: you apply it, it feels great, but it all comes off at the end of the day. You might not wear it all the time, and how far it can take you will vary from person to person, skill set and product selection. Ultimately, the quicker the hit, the quicker the fall. Apply a new lipstick and yes – it looks amazing for the first hour, but over time it needs reapplying, over and over again. It gives you that rush of surface-level confidence, but does the lipstick have the power to light up your insides and make you feel truly present and alive? I highly doubt it. A lifelong glow up is something that I have consciously chosen to be on, a want to better myself every day, a desire to focus on personal development with the aim of not wasting my existence. I hope you'll join me as our journeys overlap!

Doing the inner work can be tough, as it definitely requires a level of self-discipline and accountability. As I gradually became aware of how much I loathed myself, my sadness turned into determination. It was up to me to take control; it wasn't going to just happen! I wanted to change my life and I had to use the pain from the past as fuel to get the wheels in motion. Right now, it might feel like you're all knotted up and tangled inside; you want to unpack moments in your brain, bring it all out and repack it neatly, but it feels too hard. I too felt that unravelling it all was impossible, and that my past would always be there, scrambling my brain. It was easier to stay in a mess than do the work – or so I once thought.

You *can* do it. The inner work, when we consciously recognise and bring an awareness into how we operate in who we are, is always worth doing. Rather than subconsciously living a life that isn't bringing us feelings of enlightenment, we can begin to build a framework that brings us fulfilment.

SELF-CHECK-IN

Remember, this isn't a quick fix. This is more than lipstick. Something has brought *The Confidence Ritual* into your life, and for want of a better phrase – it's now or never, bitch.

As you begin to bring in that awareness, ask yourself, and perhaps journal the answers to, some important questions:

> *Why am I doing this? For example – I want to feel confident at work, or I want to prioritise myself more, or perhaps I want to feel my best on [insert date].*
> *How can I change my life to bring me more joy?*
> *Do I desire more confidence and can this be part of my plan?*
> *What about my life is currently raising my inner vibration, or what about my day-to-day isn't feeling right?*
> *Who is impacting my overall mood and how can I navigate this in order to preserve my own inner vibe?*

THE ART OF LIVING

Oscar Wilde said, 'To live is the rarest thing in the world. Most people exist, that is all.' Growing up in the north of England in the nineties and noughties, living meant living for the weekend! 'Saturday night, jeans on tight'. There's getting ready for a night out ... and then there's 'Northern-style' getting ready! What some may deem the decadent art of vanity is to me a cathartic process, adding to the layers of excitement in anticipation of the weekend – getting ready is about putting on an armour, making yourself feel confident for those moments where, without it, you might not feel your best.

A true Northerner starts getting ready for Saturday night on Tuesday. It's something I still do every week (although I haven't lived in the north of England for more than fifteen years, my northern roots and beauty traditions will never leave me). Stripping off the previous weekend's self-tan, booking treatments, planning outfits and choosing the right fragrance – enjoying the general process of picking myself up! Of course, this isn't an essential part of the day-to-day, but it does fall under the category of glow up.

I often say my favourite part of a night out or special occasion is getting ready. Perhaps that's why I was destined for a career in the beauty industry – my career and monthly pay cheque result from being part of the getting-ready process for others! Getting ready – whether you're bronzing for the red carpet or picking an outfit for a birthday dinner – all comes down to logistics, repetition and organisation. Logistics are how to get you from A to Z, depending on what appointments are where; repetition is the skill set you've built up from doing the same things week on week to help you feel glam; and organisation is making sure everything runs in the right order and that you get to the finish line feeling together and ready.

Sure, this is all great on the surface; we can have every beauty treatment available under the sun, and while that might make us feel confident for a moment, deep down inside things might feel very different. How do we then move into the art of *truly glowing up*? Well – we have to glow deeper.

When you start to glow deeper, the glow up itself shines in a whole other dimension. I realise a physical glow up comes with time constraints and multiple layers of effort, some of which we just might not have. Not every glow up has to be physical: you can have mental glow ups, and even spiritual glow ups!

It's easy to say 'I'm on a glow up', but I think it's important to define the term under three headings: surface, mental and spiritual. I realised during my journey that this helped me to recognise why and how I was choosing to spend my self-development time, and when I was focusing on one more than another. If one wasn't bringing me joy, did I need to dig a little deeper?

Surface glow up

A short-term surface glow up might be applying self-tan, applying a new lipstick, wearing a new outfit. A long-term surface glow up would consist of perhaps growing your hair or working towards a specific fitness goal or (if desired) having Botox, fillers or any other physical lasting adjustment.

Mental glow up

A short-term mental glow up will be anything that instantly makes you feel happy – that great moment when the dopamine is released! This might link to the surface glow up if it makes you *feel* better, but also dancing to your favourite playlist, doing a workout that instantly boosts endorphins, seeing friends who make you laugh until your sides hurt or visiting an art gallery and finding peace. A long-term mental glow up could consist of digging a bit deeper, whereby you decide to start your day with positive mantras, or you look at your friendship circle and decide to take action over who is making you feel good and who is bringing you down.

Spiritual glow up

A spiritual glow up needs a bit more description here because it goes to the core of who you are, allowing you to unpack something that's *really* going on, or you feel is holding you back. I say spiritual, but to be clear I don't mean this in the 'lighting incense and lying on a mat making the "ohm" sound' mode of spirituality. I mean looking to your inner vibrations and cranking them up a notch. Vibrations are that inner feeling. We as humans are made up of more than 60 per cent water. You know that when you drop something into a pond, the water ripples. Think of that as an analogy for how we react and deeply connect to our own feelings as well as those of others and their mood. We can become more sensitive and highly tuned to the ripples activating the vibrations within us.

A short-term spiritual glow up may be as simple as tuning into how you're feeling ... really, away from the noise and chaos. Taking time out to connect with yourself on a deeper level. A walk in nature, without your technology, listening to the sounds around you, allowing your thoughts to flow in and out of your mind, can help. A long-term spiritual glow up is when all your short-term spiritual glow ups are performed on repeat. Having the knowledge that you want to glow deeper is at the forefront of your inner psyche. It's about recognising that you might, at present, be stuck and that perhaps you need to cocoon yourself, allowing this ritual to flow, ready to re-emerge after a period of deep-rooted self-care. A spiritual glow up can be an evolving lifetime's worth of work and exploration. Curiosity without judgement, basking in a gentle thought cloud of growing wisdom. A spiritual glow up flows when we recognise that who we are, right now, isn't who we want or desire to be: that perhaps we can do better for ourselves.

Having worked in the beauty industry for years, I'd be lying if I said I didn't spend a lot of time playing with surface-level glow ups. Heck, I've made a career out of helping people on their surface glow ups! However, if all we practise is one type of glow up – new hair, new nails, weight loss, Botox, facials – while we might look like our best selves, we might not *feel* like the best version of ourselves. I remember being in this place, where I'd ticked all the boxes, but I wasn't happy. That's when a spiritual glow up is needed – the one that takes you deeper into yourself, allowing you eventually to confidently vibrate higher.

GOOD VIBRATIONS

Throughout this book I will refer to your inner vibrations. So, what do I mean by that? I'm talking about the energy that is all around us. If you love science, you could say it's the vibrations of positrons, neutrons and the electrons within physical beings around the planet. Physics was never really my bag at school, but I love the idea and concept of life vibrating at different frequencies. Have you ever had the feeling that you've met someone before? Or perhaps you've been to a place in the world and thought 'I could live here', and felt at home instantly? I believe that's because your own energy matches that of the person or place. It's all vibing together.

The Confidence Ritual is written to crank your inner vibrations and frequency up a notch, a bit like turning up the bass on a speaker. Tuning into the vibrations, or how you're feeling, will help you elevate how you feel inside and in turn shift how you are communicating with others and making your way through the world. When self-love goes in, a high vibing frequency comes out.

If vibration isn't a word or concept you're gelling with – that's OK! Simply change the word vibration to joy-feelings. The aim, throughout your journey, is to raise those joy-feelings. To recognise when others' joy-feelings are on a par with your own, or when perhaps you are working against your own joy-feelings. Picture it in your mind like a joy Richter scale.

In *Vibrate Higher Daily* – a book that totally clicked and made sense to me, and one that I recommend to others often – Lalah Delia defines vibrations perfectly: '. . . vibration is the constant bridge of communication between the mind, body, spirit, and outer world. This communication speaks through you and for you – and through and for all things surrounding you – at all times.' For me raising that inner vibrational joy should not only be your *sole* focus, but also a *soul* focus. Before doing something I'm unsure of, I ask myself, 'How is this action going to affect my vibration? How is this conversation or interaction, or maybe action towards myself, shifting what's happening in the future?'

You may have heard the phrase 'present self protects future self' – the actions you choose to make each day have a knock-on effect to your tomorrow. Spiritual glow ups bring with them a level of awareness: is this moment going to have an effect on my journey, could this act change my destiny? This awareness of your present self in turn begins a short-term glow up, which, when done on repeat, helps with a long-lasting glow up.

Maybe you're not where you thought you'd be; perhaps the journey has taken a course that you couldn't predict. You might be in a life that you didn't expect to be living. That's OK. If you don't like this life, you have the power to shift the energy within it: how you respond, how you react, how you navigate. Since creating and living by this ritual, I flow differently. I am on a constant spiritual glow up and it feels good. Great, in fact! This is your journey. If something is piquing your interest, explore it. If you want to learn more, then go out there and be the sponge, soak it up. If it's bringing you inner glowy goodness, then feed that happy!

So, what type of glow up are you starting this week? It's great when all three of them can be done in unison, and the short-term glow ups – when done on repeat – become a habit, positively affecting the future you. A repeat short-term glow up raises the vibrations for future glowing deeper ... because every week, you show up *for yourself.*

THE NO-GLOW ZONE

There are two key no-nos to remember that will help guide you through a glow up:

1 **You are glowing up for *you*** . . . and not because you think another person would prefer a different version of you. Perhaps in your past someone made a comment (it's often our mothers) on how they thought

you should look? For many of us, our teenage years were fraught with body comparison and insecurity. But changing who you are for another's approval is simply seeking external validation, and while that validation will come with a level of your 'inner child' getting that gold star for good homework, the short-term change doesn't help the long-term glow up because *your goals, your desires, your true beliefs* aren't met. Your efforts go into pleasing someone else and not yourself. Take 'revenge body' culture, for instance, which usually centres around a break-up. The concept was even turned into a TV show fronted by Khloé Kardashian, saying, 'The best revenge is a great body.' The whole premise is to change who you are, physically altering yourself in order to seek revenge. Placing your worth on aesthetics, your whole motivation being revenge? This short-term goal is ultimately unmeasurable and therefore in the long-term, doesn't work. If a glow up is only temporary and done to score points from someone else, vibrations stay low.

2 **Never, ever glow up to look like someone else . . .** that's not how a true glow up works. Surface glow ups like this will only take you so far, and from my experience breed inner insecurity. If one of my clients who comes for a spray tan says, 'Can you make me look like [insert celebrity]?', I just flat out say no. My answer is always the same: 'I can't make you look like Kate Moss because you're not Kate Moss!' Genetics are genetics; the body you've been born

with is *yours*, and you'll always look like you because that's how you've been designed! Sure – every beauty treatment and cosmetic procedure enables you to make changes to your appearance, but who you'll be on the inside will be the same, so what's the point? How you appear on the inside is way more interesting, anyway.

Growing up in a world where extreme makeover shows were the norm – in the noughties – has shifted many of our perspectives regarding what's acceptable or socially normal in terms of how we look. Their narrative was often, 'If you look like how you look right now, you are and should be unhappy' followed by, 'If you go on this diet, have multiple cosmetic procedures and change what clothes you wear then you will be happier' – which obviously is not the case at all! Change everything on the surface and you'll be happier on the inside? MADNESS! You do not have to lose weight or have plastic surgery to be happy. Fact. Smart, healthy, long-term choices – always.

TRUE BEAUTY

Whether I'm in a celebrity's bathroom before a red-carpet event, or helping a client get ready for a wedding, or teaching followers online how to apply the perfect self-tan or my favourite foundations, I see and feel the entire getting-ready process more than most! And one of the biggest pitfalls I witness in this process is when we give in to anxiety and worrying what other people will think. Rather than the run-up being based around fun and inner joy, instead it is filled with punishment, comparison and deprivation.

This in turn removes the feel-good uplifting side of getting ready and replaces the day-to-day process with negative emotions and energy. If you're prone to this (and I've been there) ask yourself what's the point? Rather than choosing fun and empowerment, you're actively choosing to put yourself through a negative process. Why do that to yourself? Choosing sadness over joy? The opinion of another person is irrelevant to your existence. You'll never hear what everyone is thinking, so why create a monologue in your head that doesn't exist? You won't know what others think … and if people talk about you behind your back, are they really the type of people you want to have anything to do with? It says more about them than it does about you, babes!

Surface-level short-term glow ups aren't negative. They have a vital role in bridging the gap between mental glow ups, spiritual glow ups and our overall vibration. Surface-level glow ups really help the dialogue in our head to stay positive, because we like what we see in the mirror. As we do the inner work, don't neglect the outside! Keep doing what you do in order to feel your best. Have I stopped self-tanning because I've learned to vibrate higher? No way! It all flows in unison. That lovely feeling on opening a new beauty product, its smell, its texture, the hopeful moment you have as you apply it – we LOVE this … but it will feel even better when the mental vibration is in a state of calm flow.

Our skin texture, our natural contour, the shape of our physical being … all is a canvas for natural play. We don't have to neglect this. If Cleopatra was bathing in goat's milk, babe, you can enjoy the beautification process too. But choosing to get ready and putting pressure on yourself to look a certain way for the perceived approval of others will not make you truly happy – you have to do it for YOU. Allowing yourself to be ruled by deprivation and a negative inner dialogue will not bring you joy. If you speak beauty, an inner glow up is the best primer for all the other beauty treatments. An inner glow helps everything on the surface act a little brighter and last longer. It's cost-effective – an inner glow up makes your outer glow products perform better. You don't need as many products to 'cover up' because you've accepted and embraced what's there natu-rally, and a bit of hard work now may save you money in the long run. How about that?!

GLOW UP CHECKLIST

Something to work towards, a goal, is always beneficial. It can keep us on track, and I'm a fan of that. Inner accountability. The goal doesn't have to be something like weight loss. It can be that by a certain date you simply want to *feel better.* Perhaps it's an interview, a reunion or a big family event you're going to work towards. Life is one big glow up if you choose it to be.

Asking yourself, 'How is this going to make me *feel?'* will be one of the glow-up checklist questions you'll keep revisiting time and time again and hopefully forever, because all it will bring is positivity and feel-good vibes! You can come back to these lists time and time again, whenever you need a new glow up, an altered glow up or a higher-level glow up.

Surface glow up
- Get a haircut.
- Have a nail treatment.
- Apply your self-tan.
- Shop your wardrobe and wear something you haven't worn in ages.
- Enjoy a massage.
- Exfoliate.
- Wear an old fragrance that brings back good memories.

Mental glow up
- Play your favourite playlist and dance around your kitchen.
- Schedule in mental-health breaks through the week.
- Cut back on your screen time.
- Complete tasks so your head feels clearer.
- Exercise to clear mental fog and release endorphins.
- Meditate.
- Hang out with and hug your friends.
- Seek professional therapy or life coaching.
- Cook a delicious meal for someone you love.

Spiritual glow up
- Practise gratitude – write down one thing you're grateful for each day.
- Nature bathe – go outside and spend time in nature.
- Create a vision board and practise manifestation.
- Explore your spiritual beliefs.
- Read motivational books.

LIKE A PRAYER?

Spirituality comes in many different formats, and every system or belief has its own validation, importance and purpose. Whatever you believe or don't believe in is absolutely OK. It's your life! If your prayer involves visiting a physical place of worship and being quiet while communicating with a higher being or deity then you may wish to bring that more into your weekly practice. Focus on what makes you feel good, what's bringing you a sense of calm and purpose. If that particular form of spiritual routine isn't giving you what you need, you could build it into another format – such as time at home creating vision boards and practising gratitude.

If you feel a calling to something, why not explore it? I was raised as a Christian, not strictly at home with my family, but I went to schools that practised Christian traditions. As I grew older, there were and still are many aspects of Christianity that I do *and* don't agree with or believe in – it just wasn't connecting with how I felt inside. I began to take myself on a spiritual journey of exploration, seeing what felt good as I delved deeper. A spiritual journey is a path that I believe we travel on alone. We may have guidance from others, but ultimately it's our own journey of self-discovery.

As a spray tanner, I found that nudity became not only an empowering place for my clients to be in physically, but also a space where truth was spoken. I had (and still have) multiple conversations with clients about spirituality, beliefs and higher beings. I find these discussions interesting, and it opens up a true level of listening and understanding without judgement, because everyone has their right to believe what they choose to believe.

I use tarot as a form of tuning into what my instinct is telling me. Many people think tarot is a prediction of the future – it isn't. Tarot presents a situation, and it's how we respond to that situation that helps tell us what we truly want. Fear can really rule our heads when it comes to spiritual practice but, remember, you control the decks. It's up to you how you view a situation, whether you choose to see it as a guide, or whether it doesn't line up with you and your brand DNA. I find divination extremely useful when I'm feeling lost. I'm the person who takes notes from the lunar cycles, my house is covered in crystals and I really believe in zodiac energy. (Despite all this I, of course, married an atheist!)

You do not need to believe in a higher being to practise gratitude, create goals or spend time in nature. If you're feeling curious towards any form of high being spirituality, my recommendation would always be: lean in. Listen out for what your soul is craving.

2

Sorting Out Self-esteem

As I've said, the clearest route to becoming more confident lies within the multi-layered types of glow up: surface, mental and spiritual. When these three forms of glow up are activated and are flowing in abundant unison, our self-esteem rises. Self-esteem is how we view ourselves and our actions. Confident people would typically say their self-esteem is high, while those with low confidence would recognise their self-esteem as low. By focusing our actions on our self-esteem, and bringing it to the top of our priority list, we increase our confidence.

Sometimes we don't realise the negative state of mind we're stuck in until someone else points it out. We think we're doing just fine; we think we're in control; but in reality, our low self-esteem may be in control of us. Perhaps every time something bad happens you default to negative – potentially a place of comfort. The predominant cause of you staying in the same place may be your low self-esteem and how you view yourself. When the chips are down, we don't move up: we stay put. We don't count our blessings, we don't practise gratitude; life just bobs along, with no great peaks or troughs.

Change is the only constant throughout life, yet so many people fear it. While it might feel scary, change is growth and resisting it and falling back into your old patterns will only slow down your growth. Those who fear change may not be confident or clear about who they are on the inside – and here lies room for an inner glow up! By consciously starting a multi-level glow up, your self-esteem will have no choice but to increase. Imagine if, as you finish reading this book, your whole landscape shifts – what route might you take? You have the power right now to change your life for where you truly want it to be!

BURNT TOAST

An old theory goes that if you burn your toast in the morning, your day invariably runs late and is ruined. What if, rather than focusing your energy negatively on the fact that you burnt your toast and either had to spend time scraping it or starting again, you start to think that the extra time it takes to sort it out isn't a bad thing. That the bread was in fact *meant to be burnt*, sending your day in a different direction. This leads me to give you one of my all-time favourite affirmations: *I am exactly where I am supposed to be.*

I say this to myself every single day. When things take an unexpected turn – perhaps life hits a trough, or someone behaves in a negative way towards me – I remind myself that this is happening for a reason. I suffered with low self-esteem for twenty years and truly understand how it feels to be in that place. What I chose to wear, who I spent my time with, where I chose to visit and why I chose to go there were all affected by my inner dialogue. I wore clothes that hid the parts of my body I hated, I spent time with people who didn't respect me, I visited places where I knew no one would say anything negative to me, or only went there because other people told me to. I wasn't in control of my life: my low self-esteem was.

I never thought I'd buy a house, get married, work on some of the biggest TV shows, spray tan some of the world's most famous bottoms, create a best-selling household beauty brand or teach other people how to be more confident. I never thought I'd write this book! But the moment I stopped saying, 'I can't' and started saying 'Why not?!', my self-esteem and life began to shift for the better. Why not step into my power? Why not glow up?

Dr Richard Wiseman, author of *The Luck Factor*, states that, 'Lucky people employ various psychological techniques to cope with, and often even thrive upon, the ill fortune that comes their way. For example, they spontaneously imagine how things could have been worse, do not dwell on their ill fortune, and take control of the situation.' I like that. So, whether you're superstitious or not, can you begin to visualise yourself as lucky? Have the moments that have felt unlucky perhaps been sent to show you that you can overcome even the grimmest of scenarios? If we take a leaf out of Dr Richard Wiseman's theory, can you begin to focus on the positive outcome over the negative situation?

When the time came to exit Isle of Paradise it wasn't a thought that came to me overnight. I had known deep down that my journey was reaching an end. Choosing to walk away from a brand I co-founded wasn't an easy decision, but I had to think about where and who I wanted to be in the future. It felt like I wasn't growing and glowing any more within myself. I remember hearing chef and TV personality Jamie Oliver saying at a press day 'being slightly uncomfortable in work is a good thing, it means we push ourselves to get something we really want'. It was a huge light bulb moment for me. While break-ups or endings happen to us all, it can be tough to process. Break-ups can feel like a form of rejection. Something out of our hands may have taken us in a direction we didn't anticipate, which, in turn, causes the situation to change. Break-ups come in all forms: career, love life, even friendships. Take it from me, rejection is redirection. Doors close but others really do open. In these times I find practising gratitude extremely helpful. Before I exited, I wrote a gratitude list to Isle of Paradise. That way, when the day came, I felt content. It helped me focus on all the goodness that I'd experienced and enabled me to move forward with a positive mindset. I wish I'd done that before some of my other break-ups!

You can link a negative or hard experience to your gratitude practice. As you write your gratitude list (your 'love letter to me' on page 137) as part of your mental glow up, are there any points on there that you would consider luck? Did you meet someone by chance? Did you spot the perfect outfit for an upcoming occasion when you were out for a jog? Did you burn the toast this morning and catch your favourite song on the radio while you were waiting for your delayed breakfast? Superstition, luck, or just plain chance – a situation or scenario stays the same, but the way you view it can change, ultimately having a knock-on effect on how you view the rest of the processes that unfold. Do you feel lucky?

Today, when I get ready, I enjoy the process. I practise gratitude, repeating the affirmation *I am exactly where I am supposed to be* as I look in the mirror. If my negative inner voice comes in and starts picking apart my appearance, I tell myself it's all about what I have to say, rather than how I look when I say it. I'm lucky to leave my house every day! I'm grateful to experience life in the way that I am. I'm grateful to be able to visit places I want to be, in the company of people I am lucky enough to choose. I wear the clothes I want to wear, and I proudly exude confidence. I am confident because I choose to be confident. I am confident because I am grateful to all of my life experiences for getting me to the place I am at. *I am exactly where I am supposed to be.*

Confidence is an energy, not a skill set. We all have the power to conjure our inner confident self – it sometimes just needs to be taught and learned! But becoming the most confident person you've ever met, and living your everyday life, are two different things. For example, do I want to be as confident as Beyoncé on stage? Sure! BUT does Beyoncé live the life I lead? No. Unlike Beyoncé, I don't have any experience (or talent) in dancing, singing and being a global superstar! I don't have the life history or set-up that Beyoncé has, so why compare myself? How you measure your confidence is based on *your* track record, not anyone else's. Focus on becoming a more confident version of yourself, not on reaching the same level of confidence as someone else. Raising our self-esteem to feel better about ourselves as we get ready for a friend's birthday party, as we try on clothes in a fitting room, as we stand waiting for our kids at the school gates and attempt small talk with other parents, as we walk into a job interview – that's what we need.

Inner confidence doesn't mean being a performer, show-off or extrovert. It means believing you CAN do anything you want and that who you are, as you are, is good enough . . . great, even! You don't have to walk out on stage in front of tens of thousands of screaming fans, but you *can* shut your front door without feelings of shame, or a negative inner dialogue.

Low self-esteem usually occurs after a series of events, triggers or moments where our inner confidence has been knocked. I was bullied all through school, for both my sexuality and my weight. I still remember a time I was coming out of a sweet shop with my mum and someone said to me, as I reached my hand into a bag of sweets, 'Don't you think you've had enough of those?' I was heartbroken. Ashamed. I cried, put the sweets in the bin and my day was ruined. I carried that comment with me for years, while I'm sure the person making the comment didn't think about it again. Maybe you're holding on to a comment someone made about you or to you?

Comparison can be the thief of joy. When our self-esteem is low, we can compare ourselves to others, looking at what other people have and presuming their life is 'perfect'. Are we experiencing feelings of joy or inner pain when we scroll on social media? Do big moments in our friend's life evoke feelings of celebration, or feelings of jealousy? 'Shake it off', 'Get thick-skinned', 'Water off a duck's back' – all common phrases for saying 'Don't let it bother you'. The problem, however, is that when our self-esteem is low, these things cut deep. It's almost as if the punches keep being thrown without giving us time to get back up on our feet.

You could be the most beautiful, successful, wealthy person in the world and still experience low self-esteem . . . and I can spot it a mile off. I'm conditioned to look out for it. Low self-esteem comes and goes; it changes shape endlessly, but it's always a dark cloud hanging over us. If we ignore our low self-esteem, it doesn't go away; it keeps rooting itself deeper within our psyche. It affects the decisions we make and how we respond to situations.

SIGNS YOUR SELF-ESTEEM MIGHT BE RUNNING LOW

- You can't post a picture on social media without a filter.
- You'd struggle to think of ten things you were grateful for today.
- You daren't make a decision without getting someone else's opinion.
- You hold your stomach in every time you look in the mirror.
- Your feel your friends are achieving more than you.
- You don't want to do an exercise class for fear of what other people might think of you.
- You have pessimistic thoughts like 'It'll never happen for me' and 'They won't choose me'.
- You think 'I'm not good enough'.

FEELING THE FEAR

When self-esteem is low, you may be more likely to catastrophise ... and when you catastrophise your life may become restricted and prevent you from making potentially life-altering decisions. You literally hold yourself back! It might be that you're confident in one area of your life, but not in another. You might be a top performer at work, but hate looking at photos of yourself. You might feel confident with old friends, but lack confidence when you walk into a room filled with strangers. Your confidence in one area of your life could be masking your low self-esteem in another.

It's OK not to have high self-esteem all the time, or in all areas: but you can learn to recognise your self-esteem dips, how to address where and why the dips are happening and how to minimise them. I love this quote from Susan Jeffers in her seminal book, *Feel The Fear And Do It Anyway*: 'The knowledge that you can handle anything that comes your way is the key to allowing yourself to take risks ... security is not having things; it's handling things.'

Do you ever have those moments before doing exercise where you really can't be bothered? Maybe you've booked an early class and you wake up and think, 'No, not today', and fall back to sleep, or perhaps you've booked a class at 6 p.m. which you dread all day. There's a common saying in the fitness world: *fearing the workout is worse than the workout itself* – and it's the same with many other areas of life.

WE ALL WOBBLE

If you follow me on social media, you might think that I don't feel fear in work situations. That things just seem to land in my lap and that because I'm confident online I'm confident in all walks of my life. Absolutely not the case, I'm human! One thing I learned from spray tanning is that EVERYONE – however successful, famous, skinny or rich – has something in life that makes them wobble. It's impossible to have courage in all walks of life. We'd be robots if that was the case. Fear keeps us human.

My friend Sarah Powell and I used to have a podcast called *Wobble*. If you've ever listened to it, you'll know the premise of the show was about what makes each of us wobble, both physically and mentally. When we came up with the concept for the show, I was struggling with body dysmorphia, and Sarah was dealing with her anxiety. We wanted to create a safe space where people could open up, and we asked our guests what was going on behind closed doors, about their journey so far, always closing with a final question: what makes you wobble? Answers included my mother-in-law, politics, my house being a mess, the fear of not being good enough. After recording two seasons it helped me understand that everyone has their thing, and that's OK. We all wobble.

I realised that recognising what makes me wobble and noting that it's a 'thing', not a reality, was a major breakthrough. Just because I felt uneasy in a certain situation didn't mean that everyone else did, and areas I didn't sweat about . . . well, my friends might! Rather than focusing my energy into my insecurities and anxieties being negative, I realised that having wobbles is what made me like everyone else. Raising my own awareness of what and where my wobbles could take me – not to good places – helped me navigate those choppy waters.

Before events, particularly work-based events, I get anxious. Networking doesn't come easily to me. I second-guess myself and often feel I don't belong in the room. Yep, good old imposter syndrome. I can build up an event and the thought processes of other people in my head to such a level that before a big work event I'm riddled with anxiety. The worst bit of the entire event? Ten minutes before or, as my friends have titled it, The Walk Up, when my heart races, my body feels hot then cold, my palms sweat, and I say the most bizarre things either in my head or out loud. I've learned, though, that the walk up is worse than the event itself. This emotion building up inside me, fear, is just part of my wobble. Fear can be an extremely restrictive emotion; it ignites our flight-or-fight response and can make us irrational. When your self-esteem is low, fear can really take hold of the situation.

Remember that self-esteem and fear are two different entities: self-esteem being the branches and trunk a treehouse is built on, fear the incoming storm. If the tree is weak, its branches lacking in nutrients and sturdiness, what's going to happen to the treehouse when the storm comes in? Through my work with so many different personality types, I've come to ask myself – when someone is acting out or being irrational – are they being mean or are they simply scared of something? I've learned that once I behave in a way that is treating another's fear, not combatting their anger, the energy of the space can change.

When Isle of Paradise launched, I was still carrying a lot of my hang-ups. Body dysmorphia and imposter syndrome – plus the comments and actions from others through my teens and twenties – were all sitting in my inner psyche, waiting to pounce on my self-esteem as I walked through life. My great unpack and refold hadn't begun. It was only when I got to the bottom that I was forced to bring myself up and out again. Can you relate to this? Are you there now? When you're at your lowest ebb, it might feel like it's not possible to pick yourself back up, but trust me – it's possible.

MY ALL-TIME LOW

In October 2017 my self-esteem fell to the lowest point it had been since my teenage years. I was on a night out with some friends in Manchester, on Canal Street, and was attacked on the dance floor of a gay nightclub. My life was turned upside down in seconds. I was in a place of deep shock, processing how such a physical violation could have happened. I tried to go back to work, to carry on like nothing had happened, but I couldn't. I remember sitting in meetings, physically present but mentally being somewhere else. It is one of the most traumatic experiences I've ever been through, and overnight I went from dancing carefree in a nightclub, to being afraid to leave the house. I moved away from London, stopped working on Isle of Paradise and hid. My childhood trauma resurfaced, those years of being bullied, my imposter syndrome ran riot ... I felt possessed by emotions that I couldn't control. I felt alone.

Through a client I met a life coach who told me, 'Someone came into your space and violated your precious energy. We can't change the past or what has happened to you but know this – you've walked over the hot coals, you've been burnt, but if anything like this were to happen to you again, you've walked over the hot coals before, so you can walk over them again. This will change your life, so let it define you in a positive way and rise like a phoenix from this. Don't sit in the ash.' Noted in Greek, Persian and Egyptian cultures, the phoenix is an immortal mythical bird of the sun, who gains a new life each time it rises from the ashes' of its predecessor. The attack, while it pulled apart my self-esteem, threw my life into a totally different direction. The attack turned me into a phoenix. I chose to rise and rebuild my life, nurturing and feeding my fragile self-esteem on the journey.

Whatever you may have been through, remember your feelings are valid. Think about what your self-esteem would look like if it were a physical atom. I imagine mine as something delicate, like a floating piece of silk. Our self-esteem needs tenderness, attention and care. It can't be neglected, because the knock-on effects can be troublesome. Unfortunately, external forces mean our self-esteem can change in a second, for either better or worse. However, there are tools, processes and lessons I picked up during my journey in rebuilding that can help you on yours. Your past is yours, and there's nothing you can do to change it. So, take a moment, light a candle if you want, and accept that it's done. The past will always be there; your past is what makes you *you*.

While the attack was hard to process, from that very moment my life changed. Mentally, processing trauma looks different for everyone – it made me realise that nature is a healer. I remember being on a walk with my parents about a week after the attack. I said to them 'I need to be away from people and I need to be in a forest listening to the trees.' It amazed me how my instinct drew me to nature. During the walk I wandered ahead for a bit to be with my thoughts. The path slowly became overgrown, and I had to weave myself in and around brambles and thorny bushes. The path cleared into an opening and there, looking back at me, was a small roe deer with the sun beaming through the leaves right on to it. It was if the Earth stopped moving and there, in this fragment of time, was the little roe deer and me. The deer stood still and looked at me until my parents scrambled through the bushes behind me, and it leapt off. Weeks later I felt strong enough to return to London, deciding to drive later in the evening to avoid the rush-hour traffic. The roads were quiet and the sky was that lovely shade of not-quite-dark purple. As I drove on the motorway my eye glanced over to a slip road and there, staring at me as I drove past, was a stag. My theory was proven. I believe in our darkest moments we are sent a sign that everything is going to be OK. I have a tattoo of antlers on my chest to remind me of that very moment.

Weeks after, I was determined not to let the attack affect my love of nightlife and socialising. A friend asked me out for a drink and, at that time, I was struggling to pay my rent because we hadn't launched the beauty brand yet. I was living off my savings so going out for a drink meant I could literally have one drink. As I walked into the bar, I said hi to everyone and sat down. The crowds parted and there he was – tall, blonde, handsome as hell, with a smile that floored me. We kept locking eyes across the bar and before I took my first sip, I knew I had to talk to this guy. The attack flashed up in my brain, *I could have died* I thought and realised I had nothing to lose and that life needed to be taken by the horns (or antlers). I walked over to him and started chatting. Never in my life had I EVER walked up to someone in a bar – I didn't have the confidence! The attack changed my life in so many ways, but the most profound was that the guy I finally had the confidence to walk up to ended up becoming my husband. I met the love of my life.

The moment you picked up this book, your future started to shift. You've told yourself that a change is welcome. So, whether you're in the ashes, or rebuilding, or in full phoenix mode, the fire is in there. In the sky at night there are endless stars, all glowing at their own frequency. We see some more often than others, but together they make the night sky beautiful. Not every star is the brightest, biggest or boldest . . . but they all glow. There is no lateral measuring device for self-esteem, and only you will truly know how you're feeling on the inside . . . but you're going to feel better soon, I promise.

3

All About Body

American YouTuber Laci Green once wisely said, 'Accepting yourself only as long as you look a certain way isn't self-love, it's self-destruction.' So true. Body confidence is about reaching a state of self-acceptance and body neutrality within your inner psyche. It's about learning to connect your mind and body as one whole being, rather than two separate entities working against each other. Your body is your mind and your mind in turn is your body. It is you. Totally wholly universally, you.

It's about waking up to some hard truths. Answer these questions:

Is your mind bullying your body?

Is comparison stealing your joy?

Are you placing your worth as a human on the shape of your body rather than the shape of your mind?

Are you holding on to things that have been said in the past?

Are you letting external factors affect the level of respect you show yourself?

Body confidence is about recognising that your body wants to be your best friend! It shows up for you every day: all you need to do is show up for it, too. Acceptance, neutrality and ultimately peace is what you need to aim for when it comes to your relationship with your body. Retrain your inner psyche to switch the negative into a positive. Every step you make, every effort, every shift in your thought process will make a difference. The more you do it, the more it will work. YOU have to do the work. Unfortunately, I can't do it for you. I'm giving you the recipe but, honey, you've got to make the cake!

My relationship with my body has been turbulent. At times when I reflect on how I've viewed the shape, tone and texture of my physical matter, I'm both shocked and saddened at the wasted hours I've spent abusing myself, hating myself and masking how I've really felt deep down. Can we be body confident all the time? I'm not sure we can, but it would be helpful if we all aimed for body neutrality, channelling acceptance of and respect for the shape of our own body.

SELF-CHECK-IN

As a form of self-accountability, I have a mental checklist that helps me monitor my feelings and recognise where I am at any given moment:

If I had to be in swimwear and walk past a whole poolside of people right now, could I?
When I look in the mirror in my underwear, do I respect what I see?

*Am I focusing on the things I love about my body rather
    than the things I hate?*

Do I enjoy getting ready?

*When I walk past my reflection, do I say kind things to
    myself?*

Is my day-to-day free of hang-ups?

*Is my mind being totally clear of things other people have
    said to me about my appearance?*

*When I visualise walking into an event that I've been
    mentally preparing myself for, do I feel like the best
    version of myself both inside and out?*

If each question is answered in the negative, then I know
I'm not feeling body confident, and that I need to put in
some effort, do the inner work and help myself reach a
place with a more positive mindset. If it's looking like I'm
lacking body confidence today, I need to think about how
my best friend would talk to me, and channel that energy.
I need to be my own best friend! So, do your own
check-in now. How did you score?

For most of my life, I felt like I'd been placed in the wrong
body. At school, when I looked at my peers, I felt like my
body didn't match anyone else's, which led me to self-
harming habits; at university I starved myself in order to try
and fit in with my friends; in my twenties I was embarrassed
by my body and treated it with huge levels of disrespect. I
focused solely on the things I hated: my love handles, my
stomach, my nipples, my feet, my hair, my moles – I could go
on. I look back on these times now and can't comprehend

those thought processes. When I see photos of myself in my twenties, there's a sadness behind my eyes. I felt like I was wearing a cloak of shame and sadness and I can't believe I treated myself like that . . . because, babes, if this is you now: there is another way!

As you work through this book, keep using the checklist above to monitor your progress. In reformer Pilates – usually when my legs are quivering and I'm clenching my teeth – I can hear all those instructors yelling about muscle memory: 'When your limbs shake it means your body is remembering this position! It'll be stronger for next time!' The same can be said for your brain. Learning the art of body confidence (yes, it's a learned behaviour) is like feeling muscle memory shakes every time. It's hard at first, but you train your brain to switch it up until it becomes second nature.

THINGS ABOUT MY BODY I DON'T LIKE

I believe we can't have inner strength without first addressing and accepting our perceived weaknesses. It's useful to identify the things you like, and the things you don't. If you don't hone in on the details, how can you begin to shift the narrative? If we renovate a house, it's impossible to do it all at the same time: we have to work slowly, room by room, switch by switch, working out what we initially like about the house, and what we'd like to focus our efforts on. Here's some homework:

- I want you to write down the parts of your body that you like (if any) and don't like. This may be a challenging exercise for you. At my lowest I remember being unable to list anything I liked, except my eyes. Over time, as I learned to respect my body, the page began to change, with more and more aspects of my appearance being added – and best believe I got specific! The length of my legs, my ankles, my thumbs, my ears, the kinks in my hair when it dries naturally, the freckle in the middle of my neck. I learned to hone in!

- Remember that for every negative there is always a positive – it's physics, baby, and you can't deny it!
- If you're struggling with points to add to your list, don't be shy – reach out to a friend or family member, and ask someone in your inner circle to help you!
- This exercise is really fun in a pair, because it helps demonstrate that what we see as a fault about ourselves, another person can't even see or visualise. Someone else might worship the parts of our body we've learned to hate.
- Delve deep. Go in. Get specific.
- While you may want what others have, the grass isn't always greener on the other side of the fence. The grass is only greener where you water it and pay it the most attention.

It might feel as if the list of things you don't like about your body outweighs the things you do like about your body. What if you stopped focusing on the things you hate, but instead focus on what your body helps you to achieve or experience? What moments have brought you joy recently? Did you eat your favourite meal and enjoy all those delicious flavours? Did you laugh at your friend's joke or feel the warmth of a loved one's hug? Tuning into the moments you experience with your body can really help with the 'like' side of the list.

THINGS ABOUT MY BODY I RESPECT

- My arms for helping me hug.
- My feet for giving me the ability to dance.
- My legs for helping me run that extra distance.
- Today I was able to watch the sun rise – how lucky am I that my eyes let me witness that?

I still dislike my love handles, but whereas my whole energy previously focused on hating this part of my body, now it's minimal because I have so much positivity. My worth is not defined by the shape of my body, and neither is yours. If the low days where I fixate on the shape of my bod pop up, I check back in on my list.

I am certain there will be moments where you will truly realise how far you've come. Where you walk down to the pool and feel no shame. Where you see a photo of yourself sat down and you don't zoom in on how you look. You are SO much more than your appearance. And remember: this is the only body you're ever going to get and the greatest machine you'll ever own!

Beauty and the Boost

When the prospect of creating and launching a beauty brand came my way, I have to be honest with you – it wasn't something I'd envisioned happening in my life. I had worked backstage as a spray tan artist for ten years prior, working with an array of products in my kit, and alongside various self-tanning brands and beauty brands. I never set out in the industry to create a beauty brand. For me it was, and will always be, about how people feel when they experience a beauty treatment, rather than the profit and loss sheet.

I will never forget the moment I spotted the gap in the market. I was shopping for beauty products for my kit, and as I scanned the aisles looking for the 'perfect product' it hit me: the formulation I was searching for hadn't been created yet. I met my business partner through a friend and told him about an idea I'd had, a dream that had appeared in my headspace. I talked him through the theories and concepts, the look and feel of the brand, and we soon began working on this new creation: my career as a spray tanner, bottled.

Naming Isle of Paradise felt like naming a first born! Fun fact: when I named Isle of Paradise it wasn't about recreating a physical place, it was about the state of mind you take yourself to when you're wearing your self-tan. That moment when you look in the mirror after your tan has developed and breathe a sigh of relief: 'There I am.'

Before you even get to launch day you're exhausted from all the pre-work you've had to put in. There's no income because the products aren't being sold yet, and my life felt like it was hanging by a thread. I experienced the homophobic attack in Manchester in October 2017, and launched Isle of Paradise in March 2018 in the UK. This was my 'beans on toast' era. I struggled to pay my rent, my friendships suffered because I was always working, and I had to get a part-time job as a PA to help balance out the funds. Financially the year before launching a brand is hard. Every bit of energy was invested into Isle of Paradise, and I didn't even know if it would work.

Our launch period was a rollercoaster, and the noise the UK launch made piqued the interest of the buyers at the biggest beauty retailer in the world: Sephora. When they reached out, I had to cancel my flight to Australia for a friend's wedding and fly to San Francisco for an hour-long meeting in the Sephora boardroom. Back then we were a small team, and we were nervous. Sephora, the biggest beauty retailer in the world, wanted to meet us! Nothing really prepares you for that. There is no right outfit or fragrance. Chances are you won't have a good hair day and the hotel iron will be rubbish. Trust me.

I remember stepping out of our Uber in central San Francisco. The air was fresh and a little cold, but it felt like it was going to be a beautiful day. I remember looking up at the skyscraper in front of me and thinking: this is it. My ears popped as we went up each floor in the elevator, and the higher we rose the more nervous I got. The doors opened into an office reception that looked like a scene from a film. The black-and-white signature Sephora stripes lining the corridors, the waft of fragrance, big hair, long lashes, full coverage make-up, no make-up, lipstick, lip gloss, brows for days. The energy in that building was electric. It felt like a dream. There I was, in Sephora HQ.

We were called into the boardroom and invited to sit around a big table: five individuals from Sephora, and five of us. We were nervous. I laugh now about how hydrated the Sephora team seemed to be, each one sitting behind a giant water bottle. Flawless foundation application, skyscraper lashes, brows balmed and combed to perfection – and then these huge water bottles. Heaven forbid the skin dries out! Gosh – I do so love the beauty industry.

We pitched our small brand to the beauty giants: gave them the origin story, born backstage, sharing our ideas behind each product. I remember thinking how hard it was to deliver just the headlines on each product, but time was ticking – we only had an hour. From one product to the next we ran through what the self-tanning water did, how the self-tan drops worked, why you'd choose a self-tan foam over a lotion. We had samples on the table. Isle of Paradise was there for everyone to touch, smell, pump out and experience. It felt like my whole career was being judged. You've seen *Dragons' Den* or *Shark Tank*? That's not even a patch on what we went through. Fast-paced conversations happened around that boardroom table, in what seemed like another language. It was a rush and a moment I'll never forget.

In that meeting my business partners navigated the conversations with precision, ambition and calmness. They all used words I hadn't ever heard before, and I can remember feeling so stupid. Why didn't I know this terminology? I smiled, nodded, presented the slides I had been assigned to, but had no real idea what was happening. I'd never been in a space like that before. I winged it.

We left that meeting, said our goodbyes and stood in silence as the elevator descended. We sat in a restaurant around the corner and tried to process what had just happened, before heading to the airport (we were only in San Francisco for eighteen hours total). I will never forget looking at my partners and saying, 'So what just happened? I don't speak that lingo!' Essentially, they had to translate an entire meeting to me. Explaining about the products being shipped from the UK and the lead times, when Sephora could make space on a shelf for us to put product on, the timelines on their side in terms of when they needed all the marketing support, the images to sit alongside the products in store, and how they saw the launch plan looking.

Back then self-tan was quite a boring side of beauty: everything looked the same. The retailers loved how different Isle of Paradise was! The colourful packaging on the shelf, the unique formulations, the brand story being created by an expert backstage. And as a creative I could speak about tips, tricks and formulation consistency, but I didn't speak stock levels, balance sheets, or gross and net profit.

For many beauty experts, bouncing from artist to brand founder is a natural career progression (it threw me somewhat when it happened to me). Think of it like a waiter eventually owning a restaurant or food brand, or a cleaner owning a multi-staffed cleaning company. If I'm lucky enough to have children I'll give them the following career advice: I don't care what line of work you do, just be the best you can be and create your own ladder to climb. Never stop evolving.

Working in America is completely different from the UK or Australia. Americans have this amazing way of upselling themselves without you even realising they're doing it. The Americans I have encountered love success, they love to connect people, and they work really, really hard. Americans are also, I think, naturally optimistic. For many the glass is half full and you have every ability to go out there and fill the other half up yourself! British culture is different, and although London has a work-hard mentality, us Brits aren't that great at boasting or upselling ourselves – we're too modest!

As Isle of Paradise launched, I was still unknotting years of body dysmorphia, overcoming my attack and coming to terms with my career going from backstage to boardroom. I was anxious, all the time. I struggled deeply with my inner worth and confidence. I knew I was a great spray tanner ... but a brand face, founder, global spokesperson? I felt out of my depth, I felt inexperienced, and I felt like everyone was waiting for me to mess it up.

In the beauty industry, brand founders are almost like celebrities. You're expected to talk on camera, give quotes to media, host events, network and push the brand outside of its space on the shelf. On social media, being a brand founder is just as important as the brand itself – the customer can learn and connect with the brand on a much more personal level. People like to know if a brand is legitimate – and does the founder really know what they're talking about? Do they know about beauty products, or do they know about making money?

Brand founder life is wild. Your inbox is full of requests to film content, to give product advice, create new products, test others, and fly around the world promoting your creation. So, when the Sephora launch happened, my life flipped. Looking back, it happened very fast, and as Isle of Paradise exploded, I had to knuckle down and get the work done. I only had one shot to get the brand off the ground, and I had to pick up the baton and run with it. I had to be in America every few weeks, meeting Sephora store staff, filming tutorials, doing spray tans with journalists and celebrities, everything on a shoestring budget – champagne life on lemonade money. I call that time 'My Heathrow Years', because the staff at check-in came to recognise me and I moved through airport security like a desert lizard across hot sand.

I also had to attend events with other brand founders, and there was no plus-one on the invitations, so I had to tackle the walk up in another country where I didn't know anyone. Networking at that level wasn't easy, and my mental health behind the scenes wasn't great. I doubted myself, second-guessing what I was saying, but I had no choice other than to get on with it! I put my needs to the back, and the brand's needs to the front. At the end of every day promoting Isle of Paradise, I'd go to bed and lie awake worrying about the things I'd said and whether I'd done the best I could have done. I was stressed, for sure – but I don't regret a thing.

SING YOUR OWN SONG

In August 2018, when Isle of Paradise was six months old, we were invited to go to Las Vegas to take part in Sephora's beauty expo. Brands host booths there, and store managers from all over America come to meet the founders and give feedback on what's working in their regions. When I say 'branded booth' we're talking giant TV screens, experiential marketing and giveaways. Tensions were high: a lot was at stake and large sums of money had been spent pulling it all together. I put myself under too much pressure to deliver and as a result, moments before the event began, I had a panic attack in my hotel room. I hadn't experienced a panic attack before; I've had some since, but this was my first recognisable one as an adult. I lay on the floor and closed my eyes while anxiety rippled through my body. I struggled to breathe. I felt out of my depth.

I was in the place I'd dreamt of being, I'd worked hard to get there, yet all of a sudden, I didn't want to be there. I cried and allowed myself to have a moment. My two options were to stay in the hotel room, riddled with fear and anxiety, or get up, scrape it together and do the job I'd been sent there to do. There was only one real option. I needed to centre myself, take some deep breaths and put on my outfit (gold trousers and a gold top dug out from my festival wardrobe). I needed to be the Isle of Paradise founder and stand on that booth, smile, and meet the Sephora store managers who were going to sell the brand I had created.

In times of need, I lean into music. Music has always felt like a way to connect with who I truly am on the inside. You can't fake liking or loathing a song, and I needed to hear a song that made me feel like me. I reached for my phone, opened Spotify and played Elton John's 'Are You Ready for Love'. I closed my eyes, so nothing else could distract me, and I simply listened to the music. It's my favourite song in the world. I sang it as a teenager on the bus winding through the country lanes on our way into Nottingham on a night out, I played it through university writing my dissertation, I've walked on stage to it at a conference in Australia, and later on in life I even walked down the aisle to it. Every time I hear those opening bars my skin trembles and the hairs on my arms rise. It's the song that makes me feel alive, unstoppable, and full of inner power. C'mon, Phoenix, I'd think to myself, you got this!

From that moment, having a confidence playlist became a must. I add songs to it that I know give me a boost and if I'm on my way to a big meeting – or I know I have something challenging ahead of me – I listen to the songs as I get ready. It helps me get in the zone.

KEEP TRACK

Make a playlist. Create the perfect backdrop for you to step into your power. Think about using the playlist when you're getting ready, travelling to the gym, hosting a dinner party or having a surface-level glow up before a night out. Music can be such an antidote and an amazing tool for our inner power, lighting that fire within! Think about what songs you'd add to your list. What tracks make you feel like the best version of you?

YOUR INNER DAKOTA

In 2018, when Isle of Paradise was launching in the US, our team grew and I was introduced to Dakota. She was working at a huge global beauty brand in America and was loaned by her CEO to my business partner Marc (they were friends) while Isle of Paradise got off the ground. Dakota is quite possibly the most confident person I've ever met. She exudes main character energy and her inner frequency vibrates high. When I'm with her, I feel like the best version of myself. Maybe you have a friend who makes you feel like that?

Dakota and I spent a lot of time together; I was thirty-three, and she was twenty-six. We'd attend events in New York where I didn't know how to act. I'd gone from knowing everyone in the room at London events, to walking into big glossy American affairs and knowing no one. Dakota was my US wing woman. Before the flight to Las Vegas for the Sephora expo, I opened up to her about how I wanted to get to a place where confidence overflowed, and self-doubt didn't exist. Dakota put down her glass of wine, and said, 'Sometimes, Jules, you need to stop waiting for the light at the end of the tunnel – you need to light up the goddamm tunnel yourself.' Dakota was waiting for me downstairs while I was on the floor listening to Elton John. I replayed what she said to me over and over in my head. *Light up the tunnel yourself.*

I closed my eyes and remembered something TV presenter, client and now friend Claudia Winkleman once said to me: 'Ask yourself, is it fear or is it excitement – because the two are often confused.' That one line is now something I replay over and over, before interviews, before big meetings, before red carpets that, somehow, I'm now walking on. Rather than it being fear, I reformat it to excitement and adrenalin. The fuzzy bubbles in my stomach are going to push me through this. I'm not waiting for the end of the tunnel any more; I'm lighting the tunnel up myself! It's not fear, as my body knows how much something might mean to me: my body is firing me up with adrenalin to deliver energy and feel-good vibes!

When it comes to confidence there's no such thing as superhuman. Everybody is equal: some have simply mastered the art and energy of confidence that others haven't. It just requires a bit of tuning in and igniting some inner luminosity.

LOOK FOR THE TUNNEL LIGHTERS

It's worth observing these people who radiate positive energy. When you feel like a spoonful of their medicine would help you, you can channel their energy. Remember that confidence is a learned skill, and a vibe you absolutely can channel. If you daren't do it as yourself, do it as your Dakota.

Who are the Dakotas in your life and how can you learn from them?

Is there someone in your life who exudes confidence and lights up the tunnel themselves?

How come they have the ability to do what I daren't?

Are they just simply thinking differently?

If they were in my shoes right now, what would they tell me? Dakota would tell you, 'Honey, just go for it!'

5

The Art of Being Naked

I didn't grow up in a naked house. I can remember our family home when I was in my teens, and at that time the thought of a naked house seemed otherworldly (if you grew up in a naked house, do accept my apologies, ignorance ... and respect). A naked house was a house where no one hid their body, would change willy-nilly (literally), a family of skinny-dippers! No, our house was definitely very British, all changing in private, which, growing up with body dysmorphia, actually suited me just fine ... but my husband (Dutch, very naked) and I have discussed how our household would be if we ever have a family, and we both agree: naked house.

Humans are born naked. According to Adam and Eve (or Adam and Steve as we homosexuals say) – clothes were a sin! Well, call me a sinner because my wardrobe is heaving, babes. We're not born hating our appearance: we learn it along the way. So, imagine if you will – me at twenty years old, having my first-ever spray tan. I was incredibly nervous about being naked in front of another person. I remember standing there in a dressing gown, with a spray tanner in front of me, and when they asked me to take off my robe, I felt nothing but shame for my body. I wanted to cover up, I kept trying to fold my arms over my torso, the cold air misting over my body, a stranger looking at my skin, at this shape I so desperately hated. It wasn't a good experience for me. The irony that I became one of the world's best spray tanners is not lost on me, believe me. However, I think that moment of vulnerability, with all my insecurities heightened, helped make me the type of person I am today. It helped me understand where a client in the spray tan booth or in one of my confidence workshops might be on their body journey.

The first time I ever did a spray tan on my own, I was incredibly nervous about making the client feel comfortable because of my experience during my first personal treatment. My career has been wonderful from that day on, every client and moment different – I can go from a mum of four in a two-bedroom flat in South London, to a fourteen-bedroom house in Knightsbridge for a government official, to backstage on a TV set, all in one day. My kit is always comprised of moisturiser, tanning lotions, gels, balms, brushes, paper knickers, a tanning tent, a speaker to play great music, and towels . . . so many towels!

Getting comfortable around another person's nudity has also helped me on my own body journey. Maybe I became addicted to that at first, just the simplicity of being naked; each body I saw helped me realise that what I worried about, in the grand scheme of things, really didn't mean anything. It's so much more than just a naked body: it's someone's emotions, their history, it's the burden of society's obsession with perfection weighing down on them – hence everyone's constantly apologising for their body, like I care what their body looks like! You're booking me for the best spray tan of your life, honey, not to judge your body. I loved, and still love, making people feel amazing. I think being naked with a stranger, outside of being intimate, gives a sense of release to the individual. A sense of total liberation and freedom.

When you're doing a beauty treatment, I believe that the energy you command in the room and in the space for the client is incredibly important; for me it's almost more important than the treatment itself (this could apply to any client-facing moment or meeting). It's up to the beauty expert to calm and relax the client using music, fragrance, talk, listening and – of course – touch. How I behave in the first few minutes of an appointment dictates how the client behaves. I didn't know this doing my first spray tan and as a result, the whole operation was a bit clunky. She was nervous, I was nervous, but we got through it. She left with a fab tan (I know this as she came back for more), but the experience wasn't how I'd have liked it. It needed refining.

Over time I began to really learn the true art of spray tanning. As I once explained to my friend's father (who couldn't get his head around what I did for a living), it's a cross between spray painting fences and therapy. Every tan is different because every client needs something slightly different. I've worked with clients whose partners are lying in the same room on life support, I've bronzed disabled clients who can't move a single bone in their body and cancer patients whose skin is transparent from chemotherapy. I learned to mix tanning solutions and create bespoke shades for clients, to move the spray tan gun at fluid speeds, working my way around the natural shape and contour of each individual body, and I learned to really listen. I learned how to read skin, and to listen to what my client was telling me about what they needed from their treatment. I learned that females will experience a slight shade difference depending on where they are in their menstrual cycle. It's a lot of work, it's messy, it's tiring and at times it can be lonely because you're flying solo a lot of the time. But becoming a spray tanner was the best decision I ever made; it changed every aspect of who I am and gave me wisdom on so many levels.

As my career in tanning started to take shape and I learned the skills for creating a perfect spray tan, I began to focus on making the client feel more comfortable and elevating the whole experience. Crystals, sage, empowering playlists, hand massages. I researched life-coaching questions to help the conversation become more productive for the client. If they're offloading, I may as well learn how to help, I thought! I would dip in and out of lots of different industries, conversations with CEOs, nurses, teachers, interior designers, brides, models, presenters, you name it – all coming to me for the feel-good glow up. The start of my experience was mainly, however, with the fashion industry. At that time, it was (and I'm pretty sure still is) a lot of working for free. I needed campaigns under my belt, I needed to get as much experience as I could – and that meant working on editorial shoots with models. And models, at that time, only ever came in one shape. Skeletal.

The fashion world was a dangerous place for me to be mentally, surrounding myself with very thin, because very thin at that time was *in*. Did models sometimes teach me tips for keeping the weight off? Yes. Did I hear fashion bookers tell models to be sick before going on set? Yes. Did I see that most models were unhappy? You bet. Whenever I look in the mirror, I still have to navigate twenty years of learned behaviour in hating who I am. Even now. Every single time I look in the mirror I have to autocorrect my thought process.

But working as a spray tanner taught me that a body is just a body. There really isn't anything else to it. If you ever get nervous about visiting the doctor, or having a beauty treatment, or being poolside, know that whatever you think you have, someone else has. Whatever you might think is the worst thing in the world, someone else has it more. Nipples are all different shapes and shades, breasts hang high and low, stomachs are different after childbirth, skin thins as we age.

YOUR NAKED TRUTH

I adore the beauty industry for all its self-expression, empowerment, softness and self-care. I love clothes too, jewellery, layers – darling, I love it all! But never forget that these are all accessories that we add to our final look. Our body, our soul, our own personal history ... all make us who we are. Underneath all the *fluff and stuff*, we're naked. So, let's talk about the power of being truly naked. Remember: our emotions and feelings towards our body are learned, not innate.

How do you feel when you're naked?

How often do you spend time naked?

When was the last time you stood in front of a mirror naked and truly looked at yourself?

When you look into a mirror, naked, how do you feel?

Which way is the pendulum swinging when you stare at your body?

Do you judge your body and your appearance?

Do you have feelings of comparison to others and to your past self?

Should you even bother having an opinion or feeling towards your body?

How you feel towards your naked body affects how you speak to yourself each day. Those thoughts and feelings that drift in and out of your brain, whether glancing at your reflection or analysing your every bump and scar, really do make a difference to how you operate in your day-to-day. Positive thoughts, positive actions. Negative thoughts, destructive actions. How you view your naked reflection can dictate whether or not you go swimming with your kids, or feel like going shopping to try on new clothes with your friends. If we feel off, if we speak to ourselves badly, when our internal dialogue is vibing low – our day is ruined. It changes how we present ourselves and how we show up. But what if we spoke to ourself with a positive attitude, and not a negative one? The day itself hasn't changed, but we've changed how we experience it.

Standing opposite yourself, naked, in the mirror – and really tuning into your thought process – has a powerful effect on your life. For me, this has been a powerful tool in learning how to navigate life. So how do we do it? Let me show you.

NAKED MEDITATION

Why not meditate and reach a place of clarity and calmness when naked? What difference do clothes make, anyway?

- First, put on a playlist that makes you feel great. Fun, uplifting, throwback songs if necessary. Anything that helps you *feel*.
- Look at your reflection and remember the fun you've had in your life. Jumping in the sea, laughing with

your partner or best friends, throwing your arms up into the air at a concert, taking your kids to school on their first day, holding your mother's hand, tasting your favourite meal, breathing in the air just after it's rained on a hot day or feeling the warm air caress your skin as you exit an aeroplane at the start of a holiday.

- Banish thoughts about any sadness you've experienced – let's focus on the good stuff. Your body lets you experience life – how amazing and how lucky are you to live the life that you're living? Imagine if you hadn't felt or witnessed any of those moments.

- Take a beat to recognise that without your body or health you wouldn't have those memories.

- Look at your reflection and accept that this is your DNA.

- Look in the mirror and say (out loud) 'Thank you' three times. Truly *feel* it.

- Don't let the work end with naked meditation. Get a Post-it note and write 'Thank you' on it. Stick it onto the mirror to remind you of how lucky you are.

6

Claiming My X Factor

By depriving yourself of food and living that noughties-model-esque life, you drain your spirit of its true beauty. That's why models look unhappy – it's because they're hungry. Eventually (and thankfully), I began working outside the fashion industry when I met make-up artist Natalya Chew (at that time Natalya Nair) who booked me to work on the talent show *The X Factor*. That was the break I needed in spray tanning. I knew nothing about TV make-up or about the TV industry in general, but every weekend I was brushing shoulders with A-listers. Kelly Rowland was one of the judges at that time, and performers on that season included Lady Gaga and Rihanna. I was meeting celebrity agents in *The X Factor* canteen and, little by little, those agents started to book me for treatments.

On that show I was working with a range of people all trying to achieve their dream of becoming pop stars. It was the first time I'd worked with black skin, with larger body shapes, with a variety of skin conditions. I wasn't working with celebrities; I was working with contestants. Real people with real skin. They taught me as much as I taught them – and being surrounded by contestants simply trying to live out their dream made me want to achieve mine. It taught me to listen to what I really wanted deep down. Working towards what I wanted to do, not what I thought I *should* do.

VALUE WHO YOU ARE

I think it's possible for a person to have high self-esteem, even appearing outwardly cocky and arrogant, without truly valuing who they are and what they need. Just as you value time with your loved ones, you need to value time with yourself. Being predominantly freelance for the majority of my career, I have had to learn how to evaluate my worth. From working out the rate for a spray tan, to my day rate as a consultant or public speaker, putting a monetary value on what we deliver as a service isn't easy! On one hand, you're just so grateful to be booked in the first place. On the other, we have to think about our overheads and also work to clients' budgets. How we assess our monetary value is linked to our experience and also, on a deeper level, what we think we are worth.

Homing in on your value will help your self-esteem and confidence to grow. Learn about self-validation. Are you properly validating the skills and experience you have in your skill set? Career chat aside, are you validating your abilities as a human being? Do you know what you bring to the table that others cannot? By knowing what you bring to the table, whether it's work-related, or in relationships, you will stop devaluing yourself.

When my friends tell me I'm successful, I often ask them to define success. What does success look like to you? Is success the house, the car, the career? Or is success being at peace with yourself? Is success measured by monetary value or by inner glow? Having met some of the most financially successful people in the world, I can say that I don't deem them all as being successful at life. Their lives may be full of material goods, but they lack a sense of inner joy. They vibe low. In contrast I have met others who society might consider unsuccessful, but they vibe high. The chips aren't down, love is in the air, and their joy shines from within.

I'm proud of my northern roots and often think about my grandparents Alice and Ken, who lived on a council estate in Wakefield, Yorkshire – in the house where my dad was born. They didn't have much money, but they were always happy. They used to say to me and my brother that we didn't know we were born, because we were so lucky. They'd survived a world war, causing them to miss out on so much in their late teens and early twenties. They were proudly working class and the epitome of British northern grit. The big light was never turned on, the gas fire was monitored, they shared bathwater, and if someone forgot their big coat, well that's their problem. While they had a hard life, their house was full of endless laughter, which taught me you don't need money to be happy. While being wealthy or well off enables a different way of life, it doesn't directly correlate to contentment. My grandparents taught me not to look for value in job titles, bank balances and cars on the driveway, but in how much love and laughter you have at home.

CANCEL COMPARISONS

When you look at a person you deem as confident or successful – what do you note? Do they always seem to have their life on track? Are they perhaps always well put together? Or is their life full of things that make them happy? If you had to write down the characteristics that described them, could you easily list them? This may all come down to the fact that they've mastered the art of knowing what their personal brand is. What's on-brand and what's off-brand for them . . .

Have you ever looked at another human being and thought, 'I wish I could wear that' or 'I feel inspired by that outfit/hair colour?' – chances are you have. As humans we are herd animals, and we like to feel a level of conformity in our day-to-day – it helps us feel safe. We naturally compare ourselves to others. While comparison holds an element of positive competitiveness, it can also be the thief of joy. We focus on what everyone else has rather than on what we have, which can bring feelings of discomfort and zap the joy from our day. We put all our energy into comparing ourselves to others, rather than championing what we've already got. Ever heard the phrase, 'Stay in your own lane'?

Comparison traps can happen in any walk of life, and whereas they're usually triggered by material goods – the big house, the luxury holidays, objects of monetary value – there can be physical aspects too, such as envy of someone else's hair thickness, waist size or skin texture. We all have our comparison triggers, and we all have a person – or people – to who we compare ourselves. I have them! There are certain people within my industry who I negatively compare myself to, and when I've voiced my insecurities or differences out loud to my peers, they think I'm crazy to even bother! While someone might be your comparison trigger, it's important to note that you might be someone else's trigger. Someone might compare themselves to you! You'll know deep down who or what your comparison trap is, right? The hard truth is you're never going to be that person, because that's their life and this is yours, so why are you bothering to compare? Let's try and stop ... OK, babes?

My friend Lucy Sheridan, who is the world's only comparison coach, often says, 'Good for them, and the same for me' – reframing the comparison trap to make it work for us. Rather than fall into a habit of wanting what everyone else has, to the detriment of our own inner happiness, we flip the inner dialogue to cheering on others while acknowledging that they have something that we'd like in our lives. The focus shifts from why you *don't* have it to *how* you're going to get it. From jealousy to motivation. Feeling inspired by someone else is not a bad thing! Feeling like you want what someone else has is not negative if you view it in the right way. Another person could light up ambition in you, but you might solely focus your energy on why they have something and you don't – rather than using that desire and turning it into inner drive. Good for them, and same for me – when you think of anyone you compare yourself to, what do they have that you would like in your own existence? How can we observe and note our desires and channel them into reality? We need to work out our personal brand and consciously curate a life we desire.

KEEPING YOURSELF ON-BRAND

Establishing themes when it comes to working out what's on-brand or off-brand for you can really help put the process on the right track. After building and creating a global beauty brand I decided to take the theory of product branding and apply it to myself as a consumer-facing brand founder. Building your own brand package isn't indulgent: it's a method of ensuring you vibrate at the frequency you want to achieve and maintain. You become what you desire. So, have a think right now: if you were a product on a shelf, what would be your brand DNA? I find it easier to break it down into a checklist. And when you start to make your own list, please remember – there are no wrong answers because YOUR brand is YOU!

Before we go into the methods, I want to explain what I've learned on my career journey about how the concept of brand DNA can apply to physical products, but also to you as an individual. When I launched Isle of Paradise, I knew everything I *didn't* want my brand to be, because I'd spent years seeing the faults and values in other brands that didn't align with my own. False messaging about products, airbrushed images, only one body shape or skin tone used in campaigns . . . to me it all felt so 'old school' and icky!

Beauty, to me, will always be about hope, self-expression, individuality and, most importantly, empowerment. Working in the beauty industry has taught me so much about how important it is to hold on to your beliefs, and what you think is right in the world. Going from expert to brand founder taught me to speak up, and to call something out when I don't believe it to be right.

Until you work on the brand or retailer side of product manufacture, it might be easy to overlook the work behind the scenes in creating and selling a product. The endless planning, presentations, and a life with two hundred tabs open on your laptop . . . I get it. When we sit in marketing and brand meetings, we ask ourselves questions: what does this particular brand stand for, and how will the consumer view and emotionally connect with it? There are teams, companies, global agencies and specialists out there all working out a brand's particular identity, and whether the brand needs to evolve or adapt. The employees, consultants and founders will work together to visualise and create a mental headspace where each can come together and connect with what's on-brand and off-brand – what fits, what makes sense, what aligns with the brand's beliefs. Equally what's off-brand and confusing for the customer, what isn't making sense, what's holding the brand back from moving forward.

The same can be applied to us as humans. As Isle of Paradise began to take off, I was very aware that I needed to work on my own personal brand. Having worked with many celebrities, I knew that they had teams of people helping guide their personal brand. I have help around me if I ever need a sounding board for who I am, what routes I'm choosing to take and how I present myself at work. We can take note of this and replicate whatever role we have to play in our own careers and in our personal lives: lifting our business strategy and applying it to our own lives. So . . .

Market yourself

According to William Arruda, personal speaker and leader in the world of personal branding, there are six key things to consider when it comes to setting up our own brand: your values, passions, superpowers, goals, purpose and the qualities that set you apart from others (what he calls your differentiators). Understand these qualities – essentially who you are at your core, what brings you true joy, your unique skills, the things you truly want to achieve, why you do what you do, and your signature strengths – and you will be on the path to having a personal brand that is uniquely, authentically you.

7

Get Real

Authenticity is key. Being true to who you are is one of the most important, powerful lessons I've learned on my journey, both personally and professionally. It may sound simple, but in a world of conformity and trends, where technology can be used to make so many decisions for us, learning what you stand for and who you want to be and become is a lesson I'm sure most people don't get taught. We should all stop, sidestep out of the present, and unpack what we want our brand DNA to be in the long term, at a deeper level. You are your own brand. You can take your inspiration from wherever and whoever you please. Knowing your authentic brand DNA will help you learn how you speak to yourself, decide who to spend your time with, where you spend your money, who you'll follow or unfollow on social media, and what you'll spend time doing to nourish your soul and ultimately help you on this glow-journey!

When you tune into recognising what you like and what you don't like about something, and how something makes you feel (as opposed to how you think you're supposed to feel), it can be an incredible tool in creating or curating something that works for you, and the energy at which you, in turn, vibrate.

And do note: the link between conscious comparison and your inner brand should not be overlooked. Unconscious comparison triggers feelings of inner discomfort. Conscious comparison cultivates strategic desire. Using a template can be useful not only for inner decisions you make in your life but also outer ones as well. Think about who you are, and what you stand for. Think about how others might describe who you are, and whether that is how you'd like to be perceived.

THINK IT, BE IT!

Doing this next exercise can be cathartic – and remember it's supposed to be fun, not stressful. If you need to set the right environment for this, feel free to do so! I want you to visualise what's already in your life and what's bringing you joy, and what isn't. We're going to work out what's on-brand for who you are . . . and what's not. Your answers can either be written down or tapped into your phone (put your phone on airplane mode so you're not distracted). Be specific: where it says 'Activities I enjoy doing', for example, don't just say 'cooking' – think about what recipes you follow, the vibe you create as you cook. Is there a specific radio station you listen to, or a chef whose recipes you love? If you're a visual creator, feel free to turn this into a virtual vision board on Pinterest!

By homing in on the things you truly enjoy, you will start to form a framework and base for work laid out later on in the book. We will check back in on you as a brand in the chapters about feeding your happy. While you might know what you enjoy doing, you might not realise how much you're not doing it. Focusing on the feel-good runs through the core of the work we're doing.

Pick up a pen if you need one, and get writing:

Values I believe in . . .
Activities I enjoy doing . . .
Traits I look for in other people . . .
What genre of music do I like and who are my favourite artists?
What songs make me happy?
What are my favourite colours?
Where are my favourite places to be?
Who are my favourite people to be with?
What's my favourite food?
Which people inspire me, and what is it about them that I'm inspired by?
What's my favourite vacation destination, and why?
Who in my life am I grateful for?

Now we've worked out what's on-brand, let's work out what's off-brand. When you think about a place where everything is flowing as it should, when things are all running in harmony, how are you feeling? Keep visualising this place, and begin to focus on what isn't present. This can be tricky. Is there anyone in your life who doesn't make you feel great, and you'd rather not spend time with? Maybe it's a dinner party and in your dream scenario, they wouldn't be there. Why? Do they have certain personality traits that you don't like? If so – list them. What foods aren't being served at this dinner party? At this dream dinner party, what feelings aren't present when you walk down the stairs after getting ready?

Are there any items in your wardrobe you don't feel comfortable in? If there's anything that's troubling you, now is a good time to write it down and release it. You don't have to solve anything: you're just noting down what feels 'off-brand' for you …

Are there any personality traits you have that you don't
   necessarily like?
What are the things you say to yourself that you wouldn't say
   to your best friend?

Take a deep breath in and exhale the feelings that feel knotted inside. Do this eight times.

Let your mind clear. Move forward.

Curating our life isn't self-indulgent – showing yourself attention and self-care doesn't make you vain – and even if it did, why would it matter to anyone else? If it's making you feel better and you're doing it for the right reasons then, honey, you're onto a winner. As much as the majority of makeover shows are a thing of horror (I don't agree with their methods or goals, dressing to look thinner, dieting for revenge, making yourself look younger), at their core they aim to make others feel better about themselves. If no one else is being harmed, and having some space to disconnect from the world and perform weekly rituals with yourself, your beauty cabinet and your mirror is what helps you get from A to B (it certainly does for me), then just go for it. Whatever makes you feel like the best version of you, the brand of *you* you think you are, baby, keep doing it. On repeat. Your body is your canvas. Treat it with respect and allow beauty to help you connect with the present: touch, smell, lather, rinse, polish, buff, slather, paint and brush all you like!

GIVING AND RECEIVING COMPLIMENTS

Have you ever stopped and questioned the type of compliments you're giving out? Compliments directly relate to the energy you're cultivating on the inside. Take note of the type of compliments given not only to you, but also towards others around you. While on the surface a compliment might seem like a low-level energy booster, it can also come equipped with a whole back catalogue of emotions. From throw-away empty compliments, to fully loaded well-thought-out compliments and even the dreaded backhanded compliments, when we pause and reflect on the type of compliments we give or receive they can come with a whole load of negative baggage but can also be incredibly powerful if directed and received correctly. It can be so easy to compliment others based on their appearance, and only their appearance. Think about the types of compliments you pay another person and think how many are often based on aesthetics.

I love your dress.
You look fab.
Have you lost weight?

Without realising it, we tend to focus on another person's appearance, which in turn repeatedly teaches us that appearances are the only thing that matters. As we know, this isn't the case, so we need to practise what we preach.

The same applies to how we receive compliments. One of my life-changing lessons in receiving praise came when I was spray tanning the Irish DJ powerhouse, presenter and author that is Annie Mac during festival season. Annie is one of those women who I look forward to seeing, and who I really look up to. It's hard to play it cool around Annie because She's So Fucking Cool herself. Annie flows with constant ambition without being intimidating. In fact, it's the opposite: her creative flare and drive is infectious. She says yes to life while remaining emotionally curious. Annie is firmly on my mood board of 'What I desire my brand to be'.

I arrived at her house, and she instantly said, 'Jules I love your outfit, you look so good today!' and I, without thinking, deflected her compliment. I made an excuse for my appearance because I wasn't feeling confident in myself. 'Oh no, this is old'/'Oh really? I'm not into it at all'/'Oh I think it'd look better if I get my arse into gear and dropped some weight.' The deflection of her praise wasn't mine to give out. And Annie instantly pulled me up on it. 'I just paid you a compliment, which is mine to give,' she said. 'Don't deflect what I've just said because it's my opinion, take the compliment.' My jaw dropped. She was right. I was putting it out to the universe that I didn't want to receive kindness and positivity from others! WHY WAS I DOING THAT?! No wonder my inner vibrations weren't rising up!

At first, I found taking compliments difficult because my natural reaction was to deflect the praise. A therapist once said to me that pessimism is just a form of protection. It's harder for us to open ourselves up to receiving praise through fear of appearing arrogant or seeing something we don't believe could possibly be there. However, learning to say thank you after someone says something nice to you is an important life skill. It puts out confidence and gratitude to the other person; it shows you've heard what they've said. Even if you don't believe what they've said at first, stop, listen, and receive the compliment – it's theirs to give. Register your acknowledgement of their opinion. Now I always think *What would Annie say?*

Whether we give or receive compliments, it's amazing how conditioned we are to give compliments solely based on aesthetics. When we compliment another person's outfit at an event, are we complimenting them, or the retailer or designer? We can rethink and reformulate our compliments to build a deeper meaning in the praise we're choosing to give. We bring a sense of awareness in how we communicate within this area of life. Here is an example of some compliments not based around another person's appearance:

I love how great you make me feel.
I love how you've pieced this outfit together.
Your energy is infectious.
I love how you've applied your make-up – talk me through it.
You're such a good listener.
I knew I could count on you, thank you for always being there and being kind.
I haven't laughed like that for ages, thank you for making my sides hurt!
You're so talented – I'm in awe of you.
This food is so delicious, you're such a good cook – tell me how you made this!
I love hanging out with you.
You give the best hugs.
I love how you positively affect my life.

Next time you're at an event, maybe it's THE big event of your year, try consciously to give out deeper compliments, ones that aren't solely focused on the surface of another person. Don't be afraid to take it deeper – then watch how the conversation flows in a whole other remit.

LET'S GET TO WORK

So, we've unpacked the theory – by now you should have a sense of my journey and brand, have thought a little about your own journey and what your brand looks like, or should look like, and the type of glow up you wish to go on with me. Is it surface, or mental, or are we going for a spiritual glow up?! Maybe it's a combination of all three! You should be aware of the importance of self-esteem and the things you do in your life to make you feel good. The way you speak to others and how you speak to yourself in terms of praise should also have shifted throughout Part One; and if you feel like you're in a tunnel waiting for the light, you should now know that you're the one who can light it up, not anybody else. I hope there's also a newfound appreciation and love towards your body, and you've already begun to activate your confidence.

So, here we go, Part Two, and the real work – and rewards – are going to come to you! Get ready.

Part Two

Glowing Up to Glow Deeper

*'Let yourself be silently drawn by the strange pull of
what you really love. It will not lead you astray.'*
Rumi, 13th-century poet and mystic

It's impossible for any human not to experience feelings of
excitement, curiosity, desire, nervousness, fear and anxiety on
the run-up to a date or an event that holds a level of significance
or importance in our lives. The buzz of the unknown, the
chatter about what to wear, who's attending, making and
rearranging plans. We put ourselves under immense pressure
to be perfect, don't we?

I see it all the time with brides in the run-up to their
wedding. From the moment they show me their new
engagement ring, right up to the big day, most brides will
change in some way. Losing weight but gaining nervousness;
an air of tension surrounding them. When it comes to the
final spray – the wedding tan, the tan of all tans! – as their hair
is put up and their make-up and jewellery come off, and I
look into their eyes . . . they often start to cry. It all pours out.

I'm sure many wedding make-up artists will echo my experience: a bride, just before she has her make-up done, will burst into tears. All that work in the run-up – the stress and inner tension – suddenly becomes volcanic and reaches eruption point. Such a moment should be joyous, but instead it's an emotional release – and not a good one.

The same can be said for getting ready before a big interview, or a dinner with friends, or a holiday. We place so much worth on our aesthetics that the tension can become unbearable. Do we have a pimple that we hate? Are we bloated? Are we having a bad hair day? The inner tension comes out and focuses itself on something that, if we felt different on the inside, shouldn't matter at all. It's not the pimple that's putting you in a bad mood; it's the anxiety on the inside. Yep, the pressure we place ourselves under can completely ruin something that's supposed to be joyous!

Now ask yourself these questions:

Is this how you want to get ready?
Is that what the process has become?
Starving yourself to fit into an outfit?
Placing your worth in front of your peers based solely on your aesthetic?
Having beauty treatments because you have to, not because you want to?

What if you had every single beauty treatment going and looked the best you ever could, but inside feel terrible? What if in the run-up to the event, the walk up, the moments before, you're paralysed by anxiety? What if, the previous week, you're stressing that your dress won't zip up? Then you get to your event, marginally enjoy yourself but spend most of the time looking at everyone else. Someone takes photos and you pinch and zoom in on the screen on their phone, commenting on the size of your arms or waist. You can't eat the delicious food on offer, because you can't breathe or move in your outfit. Is that really what this is all about? . . . Really?

After an event, if I've swapped details with someone, I often receive a message to let me know that my energy was electric, and that they loved meeting me. I don't feel arrogant writing this, because I've put in the work on raising my inner vibrations. I dress with confidence, and I own who I am, because every day, every week, every month I am on a permanent glow up. Comments about my outfit are nice, but comments on my inner power are better. I want to know how I made someone feel, how my presence lifted up another person. My outfit is fabulous – sure, I know it is – I picked it . . . but I didn't design or make it!

There is another way to live, babes, because . . .

- The situation doesn't change, but the way you view it and yourself can.
- It's time to let go, to unearth the key skills that will help change your confidence and your getting-ready routine.
- You deserve to walk into a room, inner fire lit, head held high, feeling like the best version of you.
- You need to stop pretending that life is a dress rehearsal. When your life is coming to an end, are you going to look back and think, 'Thank God I didn't eat that doughnut on 5 March 2008'? Honey, it isn't gonna happen.

- Finding a higher purpose of living – of being – is the ultimate glow up.
- Inner peace is the most powerful place to be. Many never find it . . . but I want to get you there – and you will!

This is a practical guide in giving yourself the ultimate glow job. Your glam squad can do the outside: leave the inside to me. I want you to feel only excitement for the upcoming event or moment in your diary – whether it's a job interview, a family vacation, a big birthday, your wedding, or your Friday and Saturday night out on the town. Perhaps it's about finding a deeper peace with your body and reflection. I want my experiences to help you conjure up confidence at every moment. This is it: this is where the work begins. Right now, as you read these pages, your journey from loathing to loving happens now. It's already in motion – you're in the driving seat – I'm simply giving you the route.

WHAT IS THE RITUAL?

ritual / rɪtʃʊəl / *noun*
A religious or solemn ceremony consisting of a series of actions performed according to a prescribed order.

Maybe you've bought this book in the hope of gaining more confidence; or maybe you've gone through a rough time recently and a friend has given you a copy, hoping it may bring some light; or perhaps you've tried every diet book going because your body and self-confidence ebbs and flows and you cannot for whatever reason find peace with it. Until you begin to unpack HOW you're living your day-to-day, your week and your year, you may feel stuck.

Let's imagine our life is like a ship at sea, travelling to our desired destination through choppy waters, sunny days, shark-infested seas, following the stars over weeks and years. Now let's think about it more deeply. What if your ship is on the wrong course? What if the map is telling you to head in the completely wrong direction? What if your ship reaches the final destination and you know you're not where you're supposed to be, but you can't see any other route options available to you?

Your ship is a metaphor for your life, and ships that need to change direction can't change course in seconds ... it takes time! What if the ship needs new passengers, or a different sea to cruise across? Maybe your ship doesn't need to change its appearance to reach its new destination, but it does need to slowly turn the wheel, offload some cargo, and you, as it's captain, need to take another look at the map to decide in which direction it should sail. The ship, your body and your life, might be on the wrong track. You don't have a destination in sight because you don't know where you're going. The journey is happening, but you have no awareness regarding how and why you're on this particular route ... so let's stop and take another look at the horizon.

When we turn a ship around, the wheel has to move bit by bit, tiny changes that ultimately help shift the vessel into a totally different direction. Every day in the right direction, every positive thing you do to yourself, will have a small positive knock-on effect on how plain sailing your life will be tomorrow. So, grab your map, hold on tight to the wheel, look out to sea ... Let's get you sailing in the right direction.

MAIN CHARACTER ENERGY

The main character in your life is you. Whether you're living a comedy, tragedy, thriller or a combination of every genre going – you are in charge. This is your setting, your scenario. And this movie is happening, honey, so, fire up your main character energy and step into the spotlight that you deserve, being the lead in a story that suits you. You can use *The Confidence Ritual* as your script until you learn your lines off by heart.

As I shared in Part One, I've had to teach myself how to implement life lessons that have positively impacted my own life. I've pulled ideas from conversations with clients, friends and celebrities, taking down mental notes from the super-successful while adding to a daily, weekly, and forever checklist of tips, hacks, methods and shortcuts in how, ultimately, I could become happier. I'm now sharing the framework I constructed to help you raise your inner vibrations and self-esteem.

As we begin, I need you to remember some key points:

- Taking things slowly and calmly, day by day, is a great way to set a routine that feels doable (Part Two works through each day of the week in turn).
- It might be that you hadn't even thought about your week and life as a cyclical process, similar to the moon and sun working in unison, gliding through our sky. You need to start thinking that way now, so you can get in a healthy day-to-day flow of deeper harmony. It's easy to follow, I promise.
- Lean into your ritual – trust the process. I got you. More importantly, *you* got you!

- Rise up through your pain and champion who you are; read my words and let them sink in. If I can do it, so can you.
- What makes you different – what makes you unique – hold on to that. You don't want to be anyone else – everyone else is taken, babes!
- Remember that you control the decks. You are in control of how you feel, react and process each moment. Some days it might not feel like that, and that's OK.
- The changes you will make are designed to shift your perspective on where you're at right now, and who you're going to be in the future. It's exciting! Be excited!

SETTING YOUR INTENTION

To get your new ritual in full swing, I believe you should set your intention. I want you to copy and write out the text displayed below, inserting the relevant words where necessary. For example, my short-term surface glow up will consist of self-tanning my face, while my long-term surface glow up may include growing out my current haircut. I will glow up mentally by working towards a fitness goal I have always wanted to achieve – the things that will repeatedly make my mind feel good on this journey include being with the friends I love, hugging trees, nature bathing and focusing on what makes me happy. Take a photo of your completed intention and set it as your phone screen saver or stick it onto your mirror. Have it in your eyeline! It's your intention and commitment to glowing up and glowing deeper.

Today I begin a glow up journey. My ritual begins now.

My short-term surface glow up will consist of _____ , while my long-term surface glow up may include _____ . I must remember that my glow up is my practice, and external opinions and the words of others do not validate my glow up process. The view I have of myself is the only view that matters and I shall glow for myself and me alone.

From this moment I let go of my insecurities, I do not carry the weight of others' opinions on my shoulders or in my precious thought process. The only opinion that matters of myself is that of my own and no other.

I will glow up mentally by _____ – the things that will repeatedly make my mind feel good on this journey include _____ .

During this glow up I will not neglect my spiritual glow – and while this does not have to involve practices I do not wish to take part in, my spiritual glow up involves thinking of future me, remembering that my glow up is for me and me alone. I will remember to practise gratitude during my glow up, to help others while helping myself. I will stay present and recognise that my glow up is a journey. That this journey may be a lifelong piece of work, that failure does not exist, only learning curves. Confidence is an energy that I will conjure up from the inside out. The phoenix rises from the ashes. My past self has shaped my present self, which brings true identity. I will not hide who I am but use my past to shape my future. I will focus on my inner glow first and outer glow second. I will do what I can to love and enjoy every aspect of this process. I will be the person I've always wanted to be. Habits will be formed and I will see results.

I am ready to glow, day by day . . .

Sunday

What kind of day is Sunday to you? Is it messy? Is it hectic – and are you having to muddle through it all with a bad hangover? Maybe it comes riddled with fear about the week ahead? Or is it organised, seamless? Do you serve the perfect Sunday dinner to friends or family with no behind-the-scenes dramas in the kitchen? Or maybe it's none of these ... Maybe, for you, Sunday is a day where there's a void, a soft nothingness, a vacancy.

We've all heard of the Sunday scaries – that place our brain takes us to where tomorrow it's *back to the grind*. The Sunday scaries are filled with doubt and dread. Chances are you've felt them, maybe when you were a student or in a job you didn't love – I know I have. Is Sunday the day on which you say, 'Diet starts tomorrow', like I used to? Or perhaps it's a day where you question your career, having been around friends all weekend who seem to have it all figured out. Have you convinced yourself that the minute the weekend is over you'll be back in a life that you're not all that happy with?

Now imagine a life where the Sunday scaries don't exist. Let me introduce you to the Soft Sunday, where your day is designed to nourish, heal and replenish ... to enter your fresh week softly, calmly and restored. I used to experience the Sunday scaries until I realised that having them in my life simply meant that my life needed to change. When we have true peace we don't encounter the Sunday scaries because how can we be scared of a week full of contentment? I got from fear to where I am today, enjoying my Soft Sundays, when I started following my confidence ritual.

'Diet starts tomorrow' used to be my mantra, every single Sunday. After a weekend spent going out, being with friends, eating dinners and drinking alcohol, I'd pick myself apart and the main plan for the new week would be to lose weight. That was all I could think about: *this week I will lose weight*. My entire belief system was that if I lost weight, I would be happier. I literally wouldn't plan to do anything else during the week *except* drop inches. Sometimes I'd stick to it, other times I wouldn't ... which would lead to disappointment in myself, a depressed feeling, stuck on a cycle that felt endless because – honestly – I didn't know there was another way of living.

I was totally, fully, subversively conditioned by toxic makeover shows and a diet culture. Are you, too? Assuming that being thin would make you happy? Until you begin to unpack what we have been and continue to be exposed to in our media, it can be easy to think that looking skinny rather than being healthier should be a priority. Nineties and noughties television shows like *Trinny & Susannah*, *10 Years Younger*, *The Swan*, *Snog Marry Avoid* – they all hypnotised us into believing that happiness and success was based on what and how we presented ourselves on the outside. All the advice given was about how we should dress to make us look thinner or younger. How we felt *in who we were* was pushed to the back, hidden and ignored.

So, in this 'diet starts tomorrow' era my aesthetic was high, but my inner vibration was low. Round and round the weeks went, starving on Monday and Tuesday, something would happen to cause an 'off the wagon' moment on Wednesday or Thursday, and by Friday it would be back to square one. Every single week! Sound familiar? Now I am six years into my body confidence journey, writing these words down for you makes me realise just how ill at ease I was with myself. I sometimes jokingly refer to that period in my life as 'my previous life' – because that's literally how it feels. I look back and think *OMG who was I back then?* I hadn't learned how to feel great without losing weight, because losing weight was all I focused on. I hadn't learned how to practise gratitude, or all of the other wonderful things I now do on a weekly basis that make me glow!

Balance is an easy word to throw about, but if you're in a place of deep-rooted body hatred and insecurity, your life needs to be as much about *un*learning as it does *re*learning. Recognising that how you view your body is largely based on the life moments you've been exposed to so far, not on truth or reality. This can be the hardest bit of your glow up. Live in the future and you cultivate anxiety; live in the past and you miss what's happening in the present. You need to get to a place where the past, present and future can balance alongside each other, never tipping too far one way or the other.

I remember the moment I threw out my weighing scales. I'd been chatting with a curvy client in her late forties who so confidently took off her clothes (a silk kimono with a tropical print). I was in awe of her tall, strong stance, overwhelmed by her presence. Her life was chaotic, running a huge house full of kids and a husband, as well as always travelling for her high-powered high-net-worth job in magazines. The only time she could squeeze in her spray tan was at 8 a.m. on a Saturday morning. I wouldn't have called her body confident, but compared to other clients she had a body neutral vibe about her others didn't possess.

During one particular spray tan, we got onto the topic of diets. I spoke about what diet I was on at the time as we chatted, her arms in the air, legs bent – me wafting my spray tan gun around, misting her with faux glow. She turned to me and asked, 'Jules, do you think there's more to life than losing weight?' At that moment for me, there wasn't. But that conversation flicked a switch for me. I finally saw my cycle. Saturdays were a time for rebelling – I stayed out late, I binged alcohol, I overate – and Sundays were a time for regretting. Over and over again. I hadn't yet created a diary full of the things I knew were going to bring me joy.

The Sunday scaries are real. Unless you have experienced them, you'll never understand how vital it is to learn how to navigate your way through them. I roll my eyes when I hear people say, 'Oh, don't be anxious on a Sunday, it's not Monday yet!' because it displays a lack of understanding for the pre-work-week anxiety. The Sunday scaries give Monday a bad reputation, but the truth is Monday is now my favourite day of the week! Monday is a day designed to set you up for success (more on this in the – you guessed it – Monday section). So how do we reprogramme our Sunday to stop it being scary? Let's learn how to offload.

THROWAWAY SUNDAY

Is there anything you're carrying mentally from the week before? Something bothering you? Are you holding on to a niggling comment someone made about you? Maybe you tried on clothes and the experience was awful? Maybe your ex checked back in, or you missed your train and got into trouble at work, or maybe a toxic energy stirred itself up in your friendship circle? Bin it. You need to get it out of your mind, onto paper and out of your headspace. Here's how:

- Whatever it is, I want you to write it down on a piece of paper. Get it out.
- Stare at what's been making you feel icky. Look at what's negatively affecting you.
- Think about it. Do you really want to carry that into the following week? I don't, babes.
- If you want to burn a candle or some sage, go for it. Make a moment of it, let's ramp up the process and call in the spirits if needs be!
- Scream into a pillow if you want, this is your ritual!
- Once everything is written down (and screamed out), dispose of the paper (into the Fuck It Bucket if you will). If you're burning a log fire, cast the paper onto it! Equally a bin/trash can also work. Just make sure you say 'Fuck it' as you throw away the paper.

I do this whenever something happens and I find myself holding on to it, replaying conversations in my head, questioning who I am – it needs to get out. On the paper, in the fire. Bye-bye. Let's banish this negative energy and remove the scary from the Sunday! You are not going to carry last week's negative energy into this week. No!

SUNDAY SPA TIME

Now it's time for some positivity. Having worked in the beauty industry for over seventeen years, I've become accustomed to a Sunday spa. Of course, I wish I meant I physically went to a spa every Sunday, imagine! Alas, I mean every Sunday, I prep myself for the week. I lightly exfoliate, I wash and condition my hair, I might do a nourishing mask then apply some self-tanner to my face. I'm not doing this for anyone else . . . just me! The application of self-tan or a face mask isn't about doing a treatment before a night out, it's about using beauty to help with the inner dialogue and conversation first thing in the mirror on Monday morning. Why start your week telling yourself how tired you look? Why not tell yourself how glowy you look!

Take time with your beauty ritual, even if this just consists of a five-minute face mask or a quick painting of the nails – note that you're doing something for *you*. You can hype it up with a playlist and have a little dance in the mirror if you like: this is all about YOU.

I've had this Sunday 'me time' session religiously for the past three years – anything I can do to make the Monday morning inner dialogue more positive. If I skip my Sunday spa, I really notice the difference in my week. My Monday starts negatively and I can flip very quickly into an unhealthy conversation if my skin isn't feeling its best. Ooh, and a quick side note: self-tan works on ALL skin tones, regardless of skin shade. It's not just about the shade change for me, it's about a

glow on the skin, evenness in tone and the feeling I look like
I just got back from the best vacation of my life. That post-
holiday glow for me, and for hundreds of thousands of people
across the world, really does make a difference to the inner
mood. So, use it to your advantage, on your face, on Sundays.

HOT AND COLD

During my backstage days, I was once asked to host a tanning
masterclass for a major UK high street retailer. There I was,
standing on stage in front of a thousand people, teaching them
how self-tan worked, demonstrating it on a model who had
the most incredible energy I'd ever come across; I still think
about her often! Her age is irrelevant; I think she was Spanish,
her hair curly and her skin shining from within. Her presence
was calming, and her deep dark eyes made me feel like an old
soul had entered the building. Doing these gigs, you're usually
on and off five times in the day, on stage for ten minutes, then
backstage for an hour or so before you're back on, so in
between sessions I asked her about her skincare routine. She
told me her secret was hot saunas and cold showers. This is
something we're told loud and clear on social media all day
long nowadays; you can't scroll for two minutes without
someone shaking in and out of an ice bath, However, for me
in my twenties, this information was brand new.

She had learned about this process in Tibet and practised
her ritual every week – or as often as she could with her busy
schedule and constant travelling. She would go for an hour,
taking fifteen minutes in the sauna followed by a couple of
minutes in a cold shower or ice bath, on repeat. After meeting
her, I tried it and fell in love with the effects, not on my skin

but on my mental health. For me, this ritual is a fog clearer and inner-glow giver. But do I do this every week? Oh hell no. Truth is, an at-home sauna has been on my vision board forever (I just haven't got round to it) BUT whenever I'm in a spa, or in a gym with a sauna, I will do two or three rounds of sauna and ice-cold shower. Not for my skin, but for my mental health.

This simple backstage conversation may have been fleeting, but it lit a spark in my quest for a deeper connection with myself and with the beauty industry. The way I did treatments changed; I wanted to connect with my clients on a deeper level. I wanted to connect with myself on a deeper level too, to explore new experiences with my body. From this moment I began to develop my rituals and the craft of glowing deeper and learn about feeling great without losing weight.

This process was strengthened for me during various experiences developing beauty products for shower, bath or body – all designed to enhance a customer's experience. In the beauty industry the category for these products is referred to as 'indulgent bathing' – where it becomes a lot more than just bog-standard soap; it's about a sensory journey and moment. I learned to appreciate that the bathroom is where we start and end the day, so it should be treated with the upmost respect. It's our sanctum and, much like the spray tan booth, it's where we're alone, and naked. The shower is so much more than where you wash.

- **Morning showers** can increase creativity and help ease symptoms of stress. This isn't just me saying this – a Harvard University report in 2018 said as much.
- **Cold showers** enhance blood circulation – which in

turn helps boost endorphins (which make you feel happy) and decrease cortisol (which makes you feel stressed). Again, clever professors at Harvard University have studied it.

- **Warm showers** can help alleviate anxiety through thermal elevation and trigger our brains to release oxytocin (the happy hormone) which reduces stress, as discovered by the Japan Health & Research Institute in 2016.

Never underestimate the power of your shower, babes! Don't overlook your bathroom. Put mantras on the shower wall, keep your space calm, hang eucalyptus from the shower head, light some candles – do what you need to do to elevate your bathroom time, especially on the regrouping, renewing day that is Sunday!

So, you've completed your Sunday spa, let's action a Sunday schedule. I want you to commit to two things this week: one is movement, one is nourishment.

MOVEMENT

If you exercise regularly you'll be aware of the benefits of moving your body: increased heart rate, improved circulation, building strength and helping to clear mental fog. I used to hate exercise. Really, I did. At school I was always the last one to be picked in PE class, and later, in my teenage years, I'd bunk off and go to the park with a friend and chain-smoke cigarettes instead of partaking in team sports or cross-country running. I wasn't interested because I felt like I didn't belong.

This eventually led to a fear of exercise, and in my darkest days of body hatred I only wanted to move if it made me drop weight. The gym was an alien place to me, and I didn't connect with anyone there. I felt like everyone was looking at me because I had no idea what I was doing, and I felt everyone was judging the shape of my body. Seven years ago, I went through a break-up (I know what you're thinking – 'break-up body' – actually, not at all). I decided that with my newfound spare time I was going to teach myself to gain the confidence to go to three exercise classes a week, and overcome my fear of going to a workout class alone.

I know how it feels to hate how you look. I know how it feels to place so much of your worth on the shape of your stomach. If you're in this place, look, babes, I get it. I know how hard it is to start working out, but unfortunately there isn't a pill that gives you all the effects of exercising without exercising! So, we have to move our ass. And let me be very clear: I'm not expecting you to compete in a body-building challenge or run a marathon – if you do, good on you, but that's not what I'm saying here. I want you to show your body some respect. Your body shows up for you every single day; it helps you laugh, cry, move and experience life. Your body wants you to be happy. So why do we loathe something that desperately wants to be our best friend for life?

We've got stuck. Now, I'm going to divide the next section into two, and I want you to work towards the one that suits you and your goals the most. So, let's go to camp . . .

CAMP A – Working out is not for me

This is for those of you who have tried exercise – once or twice; the person who booked a 'legs, bums and tums' class one January, found the whole thing horrific and never returned. Feelings of body comparison, your scared inner child, 'I'm not doing this right', all creeping in. Whenever you try to exercise the whole experience is totally horrendous, and you can't ever seem to find a fitness path that works for you. *Please* don't skip this section or the tasks. Listen to my fitness pep talk before you make a decision that this isn't for you.

I can totally empathise with how you're feeling. I only began my true fitness journey at thirty-two years old. I'd dip in and out of trying to make a go of working out, the odd run here, a class there – never really committing. I believed that exercise was purely to get thin. To shed pounds. I felt too unfit to work out, and when I walked into a gym I'd feel this cold rush of dread, that my body was revolting next to everyone else's. I did not belong. You might be able to relate.

When I host confidence workshops, I'm always reluctant to talk about exercise, as it's often greeted by a change in the audience's mood and body posture. I watch my audience sink into their chairs and dart their eyes to the corners of the room. I get it, I wholly 100 per cent get it. The fitness industry can feel selective, arrogant and judgemental. The shape of a model's body in most fitness campaigns does not reflect or represent you as an individual. They promote a group of people who are simply working for the brand – and those people behind the brand have an outdated viewpoint on what fitness looks like. Even buying clothes to work out in is a drama. Finding trainers feels like learning a new language.

And on top of all that, there's factoring in the time to go to a class or committing to a workout, plus the money. The financial spend of a gym membership or on a personal trainer is a lot. I get it! I've been there! However, unlike many of the body confidence accounts I see online, I believe exercise is integral to our inner happiness. If you want to glow at a higher level, a deep commitment to your health and well-being is much more important than the discomfort you might feel when going for a run. This is about showing yourself respect. Your weight is irrelevant. Your weight and the shape of your body is not my business, nor is it anyone else's. I don't care if you can sprint 100 metres, or swim faster than anyone else, nor do I care if you have a flat stomach or curves that roll like the ocean – but I *do* care about you, and want you to feel good in yourself.

Those of you who are dog owners will know how important it is for your dog to be walked. I remember one morning walking our dog Willow and thinking how happy I was she was running around, having fun, and I knew for the rest of the day she'd be calm, she'd sleep, she'd be easier around the house. I then thought about my body almost being like hers. I needed to walk and exercise my body, so the rest of my day would be where I wanted it to be. Calmer, connected, full of feel-good vibes ... and as a result I'd sleep better. Embrace your inner puppy. Find movement that is fun, gets you some fresh air and leaves your body and mind in a calmer place.

CAMP B – I'm working out on a regular basis

Those people in the other camp might already be exercising two to three times per week, the process built into their weekly routine. Maybe it's become a bit stagnant: same class, same running routes, or maybe you're only working out to maintain a certain physique and not getting much joy from it.

Perhaps you know deep down that even though you're working out to your highest potential, something mentally isn't sitting quite right when you look in the mirror, and exercising has stopped being something you look forward to. There is a chance that you work out multiple times a week with the sole focus being weight loss. While that's OK – and if that's something you want to do, you go for it – don't overlook the joy element! So:

- Do you need to bring some more playfulness into your exercise routine?
- Is 'extra puppy' energy needed?
- Is it all about the aesthetic and not about the endorphins?
- Has it begun to feel like a chore rather than a moment of body celebration?
- Is there room to add in something different?

MOVEMENT IS NOURISHMENT, NOT PUNISHMENT

I care about how you *feel* in your body, and in yourself. I care about how you feel when you shut your front door in the morning and head out to embrace a new day, when you walk into an event, when you try on clothes, when you stand and look at your body in front of the mirror. I care about the relationship you have with yourself. It's not my place to tell you, 'No pain, no gain' or 'Feel the burn', or any other fitness mantra I've seen plastered over social media. I want to reframe fitness for you, because there is another way. You can be fit – without having a washboard stomach.

You can be strong and still wobble.
You can feel the endorphins without having weigh-ins.

Connecting your mind to your body is one of the most difficult but empowering lessons to take on board. When we feel low, we're conditioned to treat our body as if it's a separate being. To punish it. I know I've stood in front of the mirror asking myself why I have this body, grabbing my stomach, sucking in my breath, hoping to miraculously change. Telling myself that if my body changes, so too will my happiness levels. Babes – that's not true! Remember that we are conditioned to hate the way we look. If we're unhappy, then brands can sell us product that promises to make us happy. We've been spoon-fed the idea that if our problem is body hatred, the solution is flattering garments, cheap gym membership, surgery, anti-wrinkle and anti-cellulite lotions and potions, a low-calorie diet subscription – you name it, it's all there to solve a problem created by society. All surface level.

I know I've said, 'I hate my body' multiple times. Perhaps you have too. Your body and your mind are the same being, because you are one whole beautiful human being. Changing these thoughts and banishing body hatred takes time, so be patient. One of the most effective ways to feeling, connecting and really being in your body, is movement. Take your weight and the shape of your body out of the conversation. This is ONLY about connecting with yourself – mind and body in unison.

Your body shows up for you every single day, it digests your food, it allows you to feel and experience emotions – love, happiness, anger, sadness. Your body simply wants to keep you alive. Biologically speaking we are simply a combination of cells, working together within our body to keep the ship sailing. That's it. So, if your body is doing all this to keep you alive longer, why are you spending so much time loathing it? What are you doing for your body in return? Your body does not want you to hate it, it does not want the abuse, the negativity, the constant put-downs. Your body wants to be your best friend, treated with the kindness, energy and love it shows you every day.

Exercise isn't punishment. Exercise is nourishment.
Movement isn't punishment. Movement is nourishment.

If the word 'exercise' isn't working for you, don't use it! Instead of saying, 'I'm going to exercise or work out' simply say, 'I'm going to move.' Your body *wants to move*. I realise that movement might feel like it comes with a level of mental, physical and financial commitment. I get that a fitness class or a subscription to a fitness programme may feel like the last thing you want to invest in. How I see it, investing in my fitness is the best possible use of my money, because it literally will keep me healthier for longer. I'm investing my money in keeping myself alive. This investment is worth more than any other investment I make. If you can afford to buy takeaway coffee, or to buy a new outfit for a wedding when you know you already have other options in your wardrobe, you can afford to invest in your fitness and in your health.

Walking is free. Walking can be combined with nature bathing, plus walking in an activewear set you haven't worn in months brings together three of the tasks I want you to do – all in one hour of your week. Slowly but surely, the threads of your confidence journey start to pull and gradually come together. You will be literally *stepping* into your power.

This is it. This is the moment you commit. Reframe the workout, and exercise becomes movement. Movement becomes spiritual investment. This is not, and never will be, about weight loss. This right now is where your life shifts – you're going to do this! It's time to look after future you. It's time to say Enough is Enough! Right now, say out loud: 'ENOUGH IS ENOUGH!'

GET MOVING

Today, I want you to book an exercise class or commit to some form of movement in the week ahead. If you're in Camp B, book a new class or a form of movement you've never tried before. This is where the ritual takes shape, because you are making a commitment to yourself. Just one class, one session, one hour. Schedule it into your diary and do not delete it. All I ask of you is one hour. One hour out of 168 hours in a week. As any personal trainer will tell you, the hardest part of any workout is getting to the workout, factoring in the time, combatting imposter syndrome, putting yourself forward. The class itself won't be as hard as getting to the class is.

It might be a hike with a friend – maybe you'll walk that extra kilometre. What I'd really love is for you schedule in a fitness class. Not book yourself on for life, just book onto one. Sure, you might love it, you might hate it – who cares! At least you've tried. Spin classes are great because they're usually in the dark and if the music is loud, you can scream how much you hate it.

What's the worst that can happen? You hate it. You make a tit of yourself. You run into your ex. You break your leg (highly unlikely). What's the best that can happen? OMFG, you might enjoy it. You might feel an endorphin or two. You might sweat out something that's been holding mental headspace. A fog might clear. You might, dare I say, meet other people and form friendships. Message a friend who makes you feel great, and see if they fancy doing a class with you instead of heading for a drink! I try to tie in some form of socialising with a fitness class. Doing a class with a friend and then having a catch-up after. Everyone wins, and if it's the most horrendous class you've ever taken, you can laugh about it afterwards. My favourite time of day to work out is before 9 a.m.– I find that if I leave it any later I'm tempted to delay it (or even put it off). But every BODY is different, so do what feels right for YOU.

Remember, you're not doing the class to lose weight and achieve the body of your dreams. You're doing the class to try something new, to move your body because it wants to move. You're doing the class to have a tech rest from social media and screen time, and to be with yourself – you and your body. You're showing up for YOU. Let's bring in the positivity. If you are already in your fitness journey, great. Proud of you! What can you do to push it a bit further? Is there a challenge you could sign up to? Could you try a different type of movement? Run that extra kilometre? Go for it! Anything is possible with the right attitude. Don't hold yourself back.

THOUGHTS OF THE DAY

- Sunday is now about goal-setting for the week ahead and placing a value on the time you spend committing to yourself, your body and your overall health.
- Sunday is the day where we eliminate any mental baggage we might be carrying; let go, babe.
- Sunday is the time we have a moment of self-care with the Sunday spa, so do your beauty treatments (even if it's just one). Enjoy 'me time' in the bathroom.
- Sunday is the day you commit to one moment of movement in the week, or perhaps you bring a new form of movement into your existing routine. Remember to move your body: it wants to move, baby! Prioritise your mental health, focus on what's bringing you joy and channel those endorphins!
- Sunday is the day when we're setting up the week for success. Nourishment for our body = calmness for our mind . . . and it all starts on our softer, kinder Sunday.

Monday

This day of the week needs a rebrand, doesn't it, because we tend to kick off a Monday with a sluggish attitude, a grunt and groan. 'Urgh, it's Monday,' we murmur, desperate just to make it through the week so that the weekend comes round again as quickly as possible. It feels like making your way through a fog, or having a mountain to climb. But since I started practising my confidence ritual, I've gone from fearing my Monday to being excited about my Monday ... and if I can do it, you can too! Monday doesn't deserve the bad rep ... let's give her a break and make Monday marvellous.

I believe how you behave and conduct your Monday structures your entire week. And when we're negative, we're wasting time. Monday could be *the best day* of your week! If every single week, you loathe your Monday, that's fifty-two Mondays a year you've spent being mean to yourself and kicking off the week with negative chat. Eventually this behaviour becomes ingrained in your weekly habit, and you're trapped in this cycle. You either set yourself up for failure, or you continue to do everything in your power to fix a perceived problem that isn't really the problem, i.e. the dreaded *Diet starts Monday* mantra.

Let's be clear: Monday is not a day to start a diet. I used to start my Mondays in front of the mirror, picking apart every aspect of my appearance. It felt very Bridget Jones. 'Today I am going to restrict my food intake and run through everything I've done wrong over the weekend. This week I'll get thin!' Because that was the only thing that mattered.

This Monday, I have a job for you: I want you to dispose of your weighing scales. If your brain is yelling, 'But what if I gain weight?', this might be your biggest clue to date that it's time to dive deeper than what's on the surface, honey. Diet culture is programmed to remind us of what we don't have, and repeatedly places our worth on the aesthetic, but trust me – your aesthetic is the least interesting thing about you. Why not focus on what you have, what's here in life for you to enjoy in abundance and what you have to offer the world around you? What's the worst that can happen? You stop reading this ritual, fall back on the diet culture wagon and buy a new set of scales. Chances are you won't die; you'll just go back to living the life you've already lived. If a medical practitioner has informed you that you need to lose weight for medical reasons, then keep your scales, but if you're not under doctor's orders those scales need to go.

And what if we said, 'But what's the best that can happen?' By saying this you free yourself from basing your worth as a human being on the number that comes up on the scales. Fact check, babe, you are not a number! By removing the weighing scales from your life, you have no choice but to *feel and listen to your body*. When you can't rely on a number, you have to connect with yourself on a deeper level; and until you chuck out those scales, every time you look in the mirror naked, every time you drop the towel, you'll place your worth on that number. Being naked should be a grounding, liberating, personal experience. The feeling of being naked shouldn't be surrounded with negative thought.

This is why diets don't start on Monday. This is why Monday is *so important* on your body confidence and inner-glow journey. Monday is where the self-love journey begins, continues and thrives. And it starts first thing. As Lemony Snicket said, 'Morning is an important time of day, because how you spend your morning can often tell you what kind of day you are going to have.'

GOOD MORNINGS START ON MONDAY

I want you to visualise your perfect morning. Is it calm, serene, fluid? Are you opening your arms wide, stretching, hearing the birds tweeting, a gentle breeze blowing through the curtains . . .?

How are your mornings currently? If the above is already happening, then, honey, let me congratulate you! Mine . . . well, I've had to learn to change my morning routine, because I overlooked the importance of a positive Monday morning. I realised that unless I had a checklist of how I wanted my Monday to start, I wasn't going to shift my week in the direction I wanted it to flow. I didn't want my week to be negative from the beginning.

I've read a lot of self-help books, and some of them . . . well, my jaw is on the floor. Who has the time for all that? I don't have the spare minutes to light incense and meditate for two hours before my day starts. Many authors write about waking up and taking a walk along a warm sunny coastline every day, bringing in the sunrise, journaling for an hour, followed by yoga and a green juice. Ridiculous. I don't live in a country with light mornings all year round, and certainly not with reliable weather! Mornings can be hectic, and they're different for everyone, particularly for those of us working irregular hours or for those with children.

My tips are designed to be easy to follow. I'm not going to ask you to meditate because I feel like that's a practice you need to be called to in your own way. I'm not going to ask you to exercise first thing on a Monday morning because again, our fitness journey is our own journey – and who am I to tell you when to work out? I'm glowing deeper with you as we learn together. So, here are my top changes to starting your morning – and your week – in a better way.

1 Banish the snooze button

Throughout school and my twenties, the start of my morning was left until the very last minute. The alarm would go off and I'd hit snooze for an hour, then I'd get up. I'd get ready in a whirlwind and mentally wake up on my way to work, where I'd negatively speak to myself in my head. Right, let's talk about hitting the snooze button. It feels good, doesn't it? You fall back into that deep sleep only to be woken up again, only to hit snooze again, go back to sleep, and round and round it goes. What I realised is that I'd set my alarm for 6.30 a.m., but I was getting up at 7.30 a.m. – I was failing an intention I'd set the night before. I wanted to get up at 6.30 a.m. . . . so why wasn't I getting up?

I banned snoozing. I realised that if I wanted to sleep until 7.30 a.m. then I should set an alarm for 7.30 a.m. and at least have another hour of consistent, solid sleep that was good for my body and brain. I've since moved my alarm forward, little by little, and now I wake up and get up at 6.05 a.m. most days (6 a.m. feels too close to 5 a.m.!). Before I've even placed my feet on my bedroom floor, I've done something that feels good, being positive and productive from the moment I open my eyes, and my self-esteem is successfully boosted before I've even made my coffee. Fabulous! By getting up at the time I intended, I lost the grogginess from my mornings, I lost the franticness, the rushed energy, the chaotic headspace. I gained calm before my day began.

Wake up whenever you want to wake up, it's *your day*. Personally, I like having the house to myself for an hour, while the rest of my house sleeps. I wake up and watch the sunrise, have my coffee and write down ten things I'm grateful for. Can you shift your alarm clock to allow even just twenty minutes extra for you to create a calm morning?

2 Avoid the doom scroll

I've made a career out of creating engaging social content online. I've built a successful social media channel and I founded and designed a beauty brand to be forward-thinking and digitally savvy. I love social media and know the joy and comfort it can bring many of us. But I also know that social media apps are designed to keep us focused on them. I know the ins and outs of content creation, and my fingers are always on the pulse of the algorithms. I've had to work on how I use social media and find a rhythm that works for me, my career and my mental health. I know the joy and inspiration social media can bring, because I help create that, but I also know it can be a headache.

Let's talk about doom scrolling, where you sit on a social media app and scroll through endless content, some of it speaking to you, most of it not, often before you've even got out of bed. Flooding your brain first thing in the morning with comparison thoughts (aka envy scrolling) creates a desire for a life that isn't like your own, with content that might not be having a positive effect on your day-to-day. It's also a huge time waster. Blink and you've spent an hour, scrolling.

Scrolling social media first thing is not what our body is designed for, either. It disrupts our natural waking progression because it makes the brain move through theta waves (a state of deep relaxation) and alpha waves (relaxed and unfocused) to focused, too fast. As neuroscientist Jay Rai explained in a *Forbes* magazine article: 'by grabbing your phone first thing and immediately diving into the online world, you force your body to skip the important theta and alpha stages and go straight from the delta stage to being wide awake and alert (also known as the beta state)'.

The bombarding of content the minute we wake up is a lot for the brain to process, and wakes up the brain too fast. This in turn may cause feelings of distraction and scatter brain as you move throughout the day. Check your scroll first thing and your brain may release dopamine, the happy hormone. Having this hit so early, however, may cause the brain to chase the dopamine throughout the day – which in turn causes more scrolling. So, what you might deem as harmless is having a detrimental effect on where you want to be: glowing from the inside out. Peaceful, confident.

Did you know the term nomophobia?! This is used to describe the psychological condition when people have a fear of being detached from mobile phone connectivity. How do you feel when you leave your phone at home? Petrified or liberated? Do you have all your notifications on? While this may feel challenging at first, think about the longer-term results. The peaceful mental place we may be aiming to reach. Can you switch your phone alarm to a traditional alarm clock if the former is making doom scrolling too tempting? How can you build the morning routine to bring more stillness to your mind? Sunshine before screens? Workouts before scrolls?

3 Hype up your hydration

We're told our body needs two litres of water every day, and that we should eat five portions of fruit and vegetables every day, but are we doing it? Hydration is important for so many reasons: it's a staple of the beauty industry, and being properly hydrated will boost your mental health too.

- Hydration helps to gain healthier-looking skin ... that's a definite. Hydration also helps quieten the negative conversation in the brain about your skin, which in turn has a knock-on effect to feeling more confident.
- Hydration also helps reduce bloating. Bloating or puffiness can be caused by dehydration, whereby the body holds onto fluids. Once hydrated the body releases these fluids, helping to reduce the bloating, which in turn makes clothing feel more comfortable (without you actually having to lose weight).

On Mondays I make it my goal to drink my two litres of water. Being hydrated is much more than just hydration. Hydration helps with a deeper level of feeling within your body, and if your body feels better, so does your mind. Your health is invaluable, and your body is the greatest machine you'll ever own. Without your body working to the best of its ability, life won't feel as sweet. It's not about eating certain foods to lose weight or drop down a clothes size, it's about giving your body what it needs. It's about paying respect to your body, treating it with kindness, not hatred, and connecting the mind to the body in the process. Ask yourself: *What does my body need?*

4 Nature bathing

Forest bathing was first developed in Japan in the 1980s. Scientific studies conducted by the government revealed that two hours of mindful exploration in a forest could reduce blood pressure, lower levels of the stress hormone cortisol, and improve concentration, memory and feelings of wellness and gratitude. Two hours feels a bit heavy on the commitment side, but if you have two hours spare to lie in a forest by all means go for it! Unfortunately, I find it difficult to factor a whole two hours into my day so I've found something that works for me, and I'm hoping it can work for you too.

During the COVID-19 pandemic nature became the biggest healer for many of us, especially in lockdown. My husband and I clung onto those moments when we were allowed to leave the house for an hour and walk. At the time we lived in London, so our walk was slightly frantic, and we used to try and take the greenest and quietest path possible. I had always known that nature had healing benefits, but during that time I truly felt it. We all feel calmer after going for a walk. One side of my family are farmers, so when I was growing up I was submerged in that countryside way of living, nature and nurture working together in unison. It wasn't until I moved to London that I realised I needed to actively and consciously prioritise my time in nature because it positively affected my mental health.

I've found nature bathing to be one of the simplest, yet most effective, ways of bringing an inner calm and an outer glow to my day-to-day. While I love the cosmetic industry, a highlighter or brow pencil won't make you calmer. Applying make-up to a stressed face isn't going to balance the bigger picture – a concealer is literally concealing stress and agitation on the skin. Sometimes we need to bring in the inner calm so our outer glow shines brighter.

Today, on your Monday, I want you to spend thirty minutes outside in nature. If the weather is unforgiving, you can of course bump this onto another day, but chances are there'll be a break in the downpour, and you can take thirty minutes to disconnect and be surrounded by nature. So put your phone away and head out into the green. It's vital to unplug while nature bathing. Even if the body is physically in nature, if the mind is answering emails or scrolling on social media, the nature bathe is pointless.

If possible, repeat the thirty minutes outside daily. If it's a fine morning you can combine this with your newfound routine. Have your morning drink or breakfast outside. If it's cold put on a coat – no excuses. If you have a lunch break, can you take your lunch to a local park? What natural elements are near you? If your surrounding area is urban, think tree-lined streets – anywhere with soil, in fact. Perhaps on your commute home there's an opportunity to stop and take a walk. Or if you're on the school run, maybe there's a moment where you can build these thirty minutes into picking up or dropping off your children.

When you step outside, think about what you can see, hear, smell and touch. Listen to the birds, touch the trees or leaves, smell the air! Submerge yourself in it all, engage with the world around you and disconnect from your own thoughts. Allow nature to calm what needs calming and strengthen what needs strengthening. I really recommend standing still and soaking it all up – what's around you?

Nature helps us feel more present. I love mixing it up: some days I walk, other days I'll simply sit in nature, or have my coffee outside. I set a timer if I'm busy and prioritise thirty minutes. I might pootle around our garden or sit still and listen to the birds. Recently I've nature bathed at night sitting in our garden and being with the moon or the stars (I find moon-bathing a great time for making wishes!).

We know the importance of a mental-health walk, so why do we neglect it? Walking in nature helps us feel more present, our mind feels clearer, and our body naturally releases endorphins. If our mind feels clearer, what does that then do to our confidence? It boosts it. Monday can be a sluggish day – fact. Whatever you're carrying from the weekend, whatever stress might have loaded itself up already, this can be taken outside with you. You don't need to pack a bag – just step outside.

As you first start to practise nature bathing, I simply want you to be physically outside. Being present, breathing techniques, headstands and yodelling can all be secondary, and entirely up to you. All we need to do now is create a moment where nature takes priority in your life. Being in nature helps me gauge how the Earth flows. The sun rises and sets, and every day is slightly different from the one before. Nature bathing helps me note that seasons come and go, and that life is all around us. A gentle reminder: white linen, bare feet and a cowbell in hand – all optional.

5 Remembering to focus

This book is designed to help you reach a higher status of glow, and we've now reached the stage where we're thinking about where and who you want to be further down the line. If you're using this ritual to get ready for a big event, how do you want to *feel* at the event? When you visualise walking into the room think about the energy you feel in your stomach and what you're putting out ... This is what we're working towards, *feeling your best self and ultimately glowing deeper.* While the external glow is important, I want you to gain an awareness of your existence and how you're choosing to spend your time. I'm not focusing on the past or future. We're homing in on where you and the world are now.

Sometimes our lives move as if they're on autopilot. We move through each day giving out our joy to others, ticking off the to-do list for a company and doing a job that pays our bills but doesn't give us hugs. Without realising it, we may get to the end of our day or week feeling like we've achieved everything but, at the same time, nothing. We may have ticked off everything, but we still have a sense of hollowness to our being. Perhaps in our entire day or week we have done nothing for ourselves.

Bringing in an awareness to where we are, our present, without focusing on anything else but simply how we're feeling, can be a life-shifting place. I find comfort in being connected to how the planet ebbs and flows. Ceasing to hit the snooze button and cutting the doom scrolling, while boosting hydration and nature, can all help your inner dialogue become calmer, with the usual go-to negative Monday chat muted.

THOUGHTS OF THE DAY

- Monday is having a glow up, babes! Minimising the negative inner dialogue and focusing your energy into tuning into your body starts the week right.
- Remember that hydration helps reduce any bloating from the weekend and helps boost a level of confidence in our skin . . . and in turn what we see in the mirror.
- Try for one day to avoid hitting snooze on your alarm – see how it makes you feel.
- Minimising our contact with social media allows our brain to wake up how it wants to, helping with our mental health and mood.
- Sitting in nature gives us a calmer mind and an increased level of endorphins, and helps us connect with the world on a higher level. Note down five ways you can connect with the great outdoors, and try one of them this Monday.
- Monday is a great day to set goals and stay focused on achieving them as you envisage the week ahead.

Tuesday

If you've followed the Monday ritual to plan, Tuesday should already be in a state of flow. As we've discussed, hydration helps with water retention and in turn bloat, and spending time outside will help calm your mind ... which all helps us hold on to our sense of balance now we've got to terrific Tuesday, the day I want you to tune deeply into your body.

We're only two days in and you've already activated your sense of inner commitment. We're aiming to completely revolutionise how you live your life – and you're now in the process of creating positive habits and shifting how you communicate both with yourself inwardly and how you refer to yourself outwardly when you're with others. Remember: the small steps you do today will have a knock-on effect on your tomorrow! Look at you now, babes, here on this Tuesday, fully immersed in a period of growth!

GET INTO GRATITUDE

Before we begin, I want you to visualise a state of calm. When I close my eyes and think of calm, the images that surface are empty beaches, golden hour lighting, thick but dewy air, a lie-in, crumpled linen, silent gardens and cups of tea. What do you visualise? Who is there? Is there anything you can smell? What noises, if any, can you hear?

One of my favourite words in the Dutch language is *gezellig*. We don't have a similar word in English, but the Danish word *hygge,* which we're more familiar with, has a similar meaning. It describes a moment of calm or filled with love and togetherness: candles lit, food in abundance, conversation flowing. I love the word *gezellig* because it also encompasses an outward gratitude for the present.

The first life update that I want you to practise every Tuesday is about feeling thankful, predominantly towards the life you are currently living and, in particular, towards your body. Remember all that you experience because your body and your senses allow you to do so. Without appreciation towards our physical being, moving into a space of self-love towards our physical self isn't going to happen. It's important to recognise everything your body works hard for and everything you want it to achieve – like keeping you alive and getting you from sunrise to sunset every single day!

I want you to write in your notebook (or on your phone if you prefer) five things you're grateful to your body for. I find it helps to write them almost as if I'm writing a love letter to my body. Your gratitude list will probably change from week to week because, let's face it, external factors affect our mood and how we feel within our body. Change is the only constant. My advice is to roll with it, babes. Allow your Tuesday morning gratitude list to be a place of recentring and checking in with your emotions towards your body. We're all human, so don't for a second think everyone is body confident or loves their body every single second of the day. Whatever you might be led to believe on social media, I don't believe that's physically possible! But what *is* possible is raising the levels of respect and self-love you give to your body week on week. In turn that self-respect will have a positive impact on your mind and you will begin to connect as one whole being ... a bit like you're connecting the dots. Let's bring in the gratitude!

A LOVE LETTER TO ME

Dear Body,
I am grateful that you:
  1
  2
  3
  4
  5

You can be grateful for ANYTHING – be specific, be silly, go small! In the past I've written down things like *I'm grateful you allow me to taste peaches, that you gave me the ability to hear The Spice Girls, that you let me laugh yesterday with my best friend, that you got me out of bed today*! The list is ENDLESS. Showing gratitude and awareness to your body is not self-indulgent. It's a vital part of this ritual, and brings a deeper sense of purpose to yourself, to who YOU are! We spend so long wanting to change or modify the shape of our body that we forget how incredible it is. Nourish, don't punish.

NUDE IS NOT RUDE

Let's strip your next task down to the bare bones. I want you to add time into your morning routine – an extra three to five minutes after your shower or bath (I find listening to a song helpful to monitor the time spent). As your dry off your body, or as you moisturise, consciously tune into the texture of your skin, notice your scars or freckles, appreciate curves in your frame and how your body naturally indents in some places and protrudes in others. Slow down into your nudity and banish any thoughts of hatred. This time is about noticing and registering your body as it is right now, and is a good time to check back in on your gratitude list. What did your body do for you yesterday, and what can it do for you today? Stick a Post-it listing the five things you're grateful for on your mirror and keep checking on it every time you look at yourself. Allow the process to flow in unison.

Whether you sprinkle in self-love or acceptance is entirely up to you. This is about acknowledging the factual shape and texture of your incredible body. It is incredible because it's keeping you alive. The shape of your body or the size of your waist does not determine if your body is incredible or not. By practising gratitude and prolonging the time you spend naked, you begin to minimise the feelings of negativity you may hold towards your appearance and move into a place of body neutrality. When done on repeat these steps may help you move towards a place of increased body confidence.

During the period of my life where I began carving out this ritual, I repeated this process over and over, week on week, every Tuesday. I noticed that over time my feelings towards my body changed. I realised that my body was a victim of twenty years of trauma. Have you done anything similar to the torments I used to bestow on my undervalued body?

- Yo-yo dieting.
- Pulling or grabbing skin in front of the mirror with shame.
- A constantly abusive inner dialogue.
- Openly saying mean things about my body in front of my peers, hoping they'd say things like, 'No, don't be silly!' – almost as if I was seeking validation from others – and not from myself.

My poor body, desperately wanting to be my best friend, only to receive rejection in return. You may feel something similar, and it's OK to experience these feelings. Allow them to surface, allow yourself to accept that you may have mistreated your body. We can't change or control the past – it's happened, babes. The past can shape who we are today either positively or negatively. Whether your past presents itself as ego and insecurity, or whether it surfaces as a calm wisdom, is up to you and your ability and willingness to process what's happened. We carry around these emotions every day, storing them under our skin – when you say that out loud it doesn't make sense, does it? Why would you carry feelings of hatred around with you? Hatred towards the one thing that truly wants you to be happy?

Note how you feel towards other people's bodies and whether you allow yourself to be part of body-shaming conversations. If a group of your friends all moan about how they look, using phrases like, 'I hate my thighs', 'I wish I had a different nose', 'I've put on so much weight' – are you going to join in or stay silent? Joining in simply keeps the dialogue churning in your head; staying silent puts it out into your universe that you want to live a different way.

During the time I was teaching myself these lessons, I'd walk away from these conversations – make a cup of tea, go to the bathroom, change the subject. Your journey is precious to who you are and where you want to be. If you don't want to get involved in that chatter, then don't! Remember: the only opinion about your appearance that matters is yours. If another human is thinking negatively about how you look, it says more about them than it does about you, babe! Your vibe attracts your tribe – and is that the kind of energy you want around you anyway?

Tuesday will play a vital role in your journey and in your ritual. At first, I'm not expecting you to scream I LOVE YOU in the mirror, although we can totally work towards that! Instead, I want you to begin a process of acceptance, and allowing inner feelings to surface. You are worth so much more than a life spent hating your body. On Tuesdays (and eventually every day), do not bitch and moan about your body. When you go to the bathroom at work, don't speak shit to yourself when you look in the mirror. If someone pays you a compliment, say thank you. When you walk past a car window or a shopfront and catch a glimpse of yourself, do not speak negatively to yourself. Speaking badly to yourself is a learned habit – and from this Tuesday onwards, you're going to unlearn this and relearn the art of self-love.

THOUGHTS OF THE DAY

- Tuesday is a day where you turn the wheel of the body-confidence ship! You're already doing it, it's already happening!
- Focus on the five things you wrote in your notepad or in this book this morning. Whatever you do, don't cast off these emotions or compliments towards your body as the day or week progresses.
- Enjoy your body. Don't scrimp on naked time, or bathing, showering, moisturising. It's all replenishing and allows you to be more comfortable in your own skin.
- A vital part of this ritual is to recognise your current thought process. You are so capable of greatness, on Tuesdays and every day.
- Don't allow learned behaviour from society to affect how you navigate your life, or allow toxic conversations with friends to lower your vibe. This is your journey. Yours alone. Listen to your heart, babes.

Wednesday

I've always loved this quote by the late American tennis star Arthur Ashe: 'Start where you are. Use what you have. Do what you can.' These words strike me as the perfect message for midweek, for starting your Wednesday on the right note. Look around you. Listen. Feel. Touch. Wednesday is the perfect day to make connections to things that bring us joy . . . many of which will already be in our orbit – we just need to use what we've got and reframe how we think about things.

I began photographing the small moments that brought me joy and saving them on my phone in a folder marked Glimmers. Sure, we all talk about finding joy in the big stuff such as birthday parties, romantic dates, a child's first school play, but we often forget to focus on the smaller pockets of joy. If you are familiar with the term 'trigger', when something in your day triggers an unhappy feeling or memory, then a glimmer is the opposite. It's almost like a sunbeam shining through into your day when you least expect it – but, unless you train your brain to recognise it, you might miss it altogether. And think how sad that is: we miss the rays of joy shining throughout our life because all our brain is focused on is the big stuff.

Let's measure your joy level on this Wednesday:

- Can you list all the things that spark joy in your day-to-day?
- Ultimately the things that make you happy?
- What do you have currently in your life that's delivering those joy vibes?
- Are you living a life with purpose or are you simply existing?

From being bullied throughout my school days for simply *trying* to be myself, to then later being attacked for just *being* myself, my go-to thought process was always that *something was wrong with me.* When you're in that mental headspace, your inner dialogue is very self-deprecating and it becomes hard to see the wood for the trees. Life can feel out of balance – a combination of busyness and nothingness – and, ultimately, a place of loneliness.

Unless someone else points it out, you might not realise you're being suffocated by loneliness. We can be surrounded by people, yet still feel lonely. During my period of recovery after my attack I realised I was lonely, unhappy, and that I wasn't focusing on inner growth, self-progression, or doing any form of nurturing in my daily life. That's when I realised that I needed to find and feed my happy. I needed to tune into my intuition to work out what was bringing me true joy – and do more of it!

TACKLING LONELINESS

One of the greatest tips I picked up when I was feeling lonely was to acknowledge the people in my life who weren't actual friends, but whose lives overlapped with mine in one way or another during the course of the week. Sharing small yet pleasant conversations, waving to one another, merely recognising their existence and how it runs parallel to your own (without being truly in it) can be way more powerful than you think. It reminds us that we are here, present, alive, existing and – importantly – seen.

Our lives today are so fixated on social media accounts or WhatsApp groups that we're losing sight of who's in our day-to-day orbit. Having lived in some major cities around the world, I know that saying good morning can actually take people aback; addressing a total stranger in a big city can sometimes feel alien! When you take a moment to reflect on that, doesn't that feel crazy? It's just human interaction.

At the time of my attack I was living in London, a city known for its loneliness. A city full of people, but a city that can feel full of no one to talk to or have real connections with. Or that feels empty, I should say. Slowly pulling my life back together, I had a moment to think about who around me I could somehow subliminally connect with. After taking a pile of clothes to my dry cleaner, who seemed lovely, I decided to start waving to him every time I walked past his shop. When I thought about it, he had run his hands up my inside leg on many occasions during clothing alterations (the most inti-macy I'd had in months at that point – not to be overlooked!). We'd also shared multiple small-talk conversations, and his wife tinted my eyelashes in the salon next door – surely this was good morning wave-worthy? Every time I made my way to the bus stop in Ravenscourt Park, West London, I waved, and he waved back. We smiled at one another and each time it made me feel good – great, in fact! I felt seen, present, and it really helped with my loneliness.

If you see the someone every day – maybe who you buy a coffee from, or the same person who scans your food at the supermarket, or a familiar face at the gym – say hi. You don't have to be friends or know each other's big life moments – we're doing zero pressure here. You're simply taking a moment to acknowledge their existence, as they will be acknowledging yours.

In 2020, my husband and I moved from London to a small town on the Kent coast, and I once again felt intense feelings of loneliness. My days were filled with screen time – working remotely or FaceTime catch-ups with friends elsewhere, and I realised I was lacking in-person connections. I needed someone to wave to! One day I noticed that on my morning run I would pass the same car, at the same time, every Tuesday and Thursday near the local fishmonger. The driver who was pulled up and waiting for the shop to open was female, twenty years older than me, rosy cheeks, dark hair, practical clothes and always reading a book. Every time, just before I ran past her car, she would look up and see me. It started with a smile, that eventually over time turned into a smile accessorised with a wave. My feelings of loneliness slowly subsided.

One Tuesday, the car was nowhere to be seen. I presumed the driver's work had changed or perhaps she was away, and I didn't see her for several months. My runs lacked a wave, and admittedly I missed her, but I figured that perhaps she'd moved on or found another fishmonger to work in. One day, the car reappeared. I ran past and the driver flung both hands out of the window, waving wildly, with the biggest grin on her face. She was elated! 'I've been off sick from work and today is my first day back!' she shouted, with tears in her eyes. I will never forget the sheer joy on her face as I ran past and waved. I yelled, 'It's SO good to see you again!' – it was – and that was it! We still wave to one another today, four years on. Neither of us know the other's name. We wave. Acknowledge the other's existence and carry on living our lives.

Never forget you're alive, here in this world, living your life. You are a powerful being, surrounded by magnificent energy waiting to be lit up. You have every inch of ability, drive and fire within you to light up any dark tunnel. The little steps, the tiny changes, even the waves to total strangers will make a difference. Smile or wave to someone this Wednesday when you're out and about; pay someone a compliment, hold open the door for them. You're the one who can make magic happen. This Wednesday, I want you to find your lady in the silver car or your dry cleaner or someone in your day-to-day who you can wave at.

FIND YOUR HAPPY

Bringing an element of awareness into how you spend your time sits pretty much at the crux of *The Confidence Ritual*. Rather than moving through life with feelings on autopilot or cruise control, allow a moment to put the brakes on and question if the route you're taking is actually the one you wish to be on. Life is too short to not be doing things that make you feel happy. Life is too short to overlook joy!

I don't believe we can be happy all the time, and there's no happiness without sadness, just like there is no light without darkness. However, I do think we can spark more joy in our daily lives, and consciously curate a life that's filled with more activities that make us happier. Whether it's recognising that you might be neglecting your creative side or perhaps you've stopped journaling, when actually it helps your mental health. Actively thinking about how you spend your time, and what you can do to increase your serotonin (a chemical messenger that affects many biological functions in the body, including mood, memory and behaviour) and dopamine (a chemical messenger in the brain that affects movement, motivation and reward-seeking) is important.

Giving yourself goals and challenges that aren't linked to your career is a great way of keeping active, staying productive and fuelling your inner spark. At twenty-two, I decided to teach myself how to cook, for no other reason than to learn something I thought might be beneficial in later life (the language of love and all that). I maintained and nurtured that skill through my twenties, and it still brings me intense moments of joy. Cooking isn't linked to my work; it's purely a time for exploration and love. I also highly value the time it gives me away from a screen. Learning how to cook has taken me in so many directions within the kitchen. At first, I could barely boil an egg, but I figured just tackle one recipe a week, and it'll get better. I still can't do pastry, but I can cook!

Perhaps you've always enjoyed life drawing, but for some reason haven't done it in a while? Or you feel a desire to try amateur dramatics? Are martial arts calling? Maybe you climbed a mountain once, loved it, but for some reason haven't been out hiking for months? Are you making time for the things in life that spark joy? Is there space for a new hobby? Are you hanging out enough with all of your energy radiators?

SPARKING JOY

- Take a piece of paper and divide it into two columns.
- Head the first column: 'Things That Make Me Happy'.
- Head the second column: 'How Many Times I've Done Them In The Last Month' (or even 'Year').
- Number the rows 1–10 and get cracking.

I revisit this list when I'm in a place of flux, most often during the winter as I experience Seasonal Affective Disorder and can feel quite joyless and dull. I've also found this list beneficial after going through a break-up or in a place of low-vibing energy when I need to focus on the parts of life that bring joy. It's great, too, to note the feelings of accomplishment I get when I do them on repeat!

- Draw a circle in the corner of the paper and list the names of those people who bring you joy.

As you begin to fill out the sheet, it may come as a shock to realise how little you've done this month or year that really focuses on making you happy, as well as how little you've seen the people who really bring you feelings of joy. This exercise is designed to make you aware of how you're choosing to spend your time. Until you see how often you're doing the things that truly bring you joy, how will you ever realise how little you might be doing?

Life is short and unpredictable. Life can change its course at any moment. So why aren't you doing more of what makes you feel good? Isn't this what life's all about? *Feeling things*? You now have a list of things you know will make you happy. So, let's start crossing them off! Whether on Wednesdays you hatch a plan or complete a plan, let's bring more joy into your day-to-day!

Glimmers: 100 things to be happy about

There is so much joy and goodness oozing and flowing all around us every single day, and yet when we're not feeling our best it can be hard to notice the good, focusing instead on the things that aren't going well. It's time for some glimmers. I thought it might be useful to list 100 universal, simple things in life to be happy about, because gratitude plays a huge part in how we operate in creating our future selves; being grateful for the glimmers, the small sparks of joy we encounter on a daily basis are worth their weight in gold. Let this list be a reminder if you need help in sparking joy along your journey.

I suggest you turn the page corner down for this section of the book so you can easily keep coming back and checking in. Feel free to add your own suggestions at the end – I'm always adding to mine!

1 A freshly made hot drink – brewed by someone else.
2 Hugs with your friends.
3 Laughing until you cry.
4 Fresh flowers.

5 A clean house.

6 An unexpected cookie on the side of your coffee.

7 Baby cuddles and the smell of their head.

8 Waking up after a deep sleep.

9 An empty laundry basket.

10 House plants thriving because of your care.

11 Car raving.

12 A beautiful sunset.

13 Freshly washed bedlinen.

14 A clear night sky full of stars.

15 When your favourite song comes on the radio.

16 When the car-parking fairies give you that perfect parking spot.

17 Candles and the ambience they create in your home.

18 Puppies and kittens.

19 Stepping off the aeroplane on holiday.

20 The comfort of an elasticated waistband.

21 That feeling when you get home and you put on your comfiest clothes.

22 Children in fancy dress.

23 Finding somewhere totally secluded to relax in.

24 Freshly cut grass.

25 Sweet and salty popcorn.

26 Finding money in a pocket.

27 Receiving a card in the post.

28 Planning something for another person and seeing their reaction.

29 When something you cooked turns out way tastier than you imagined.

30 When a dog sits on your foot.

31 When you try a new restaurant and love it.

32 Train picnics.

33 Receiving a 'Miss you' text.

34 Blowing out birthday candles and making a wish.

35 When something you dreaded turns out OK.

36 A traffic-free journey.

37 When a grandparent curses.

38 The smell of real coffee.

39 Finding something you thought you'd lost.

40 Fields of golden wheat.

41 Anything for free.

42 Fixing a date in the diary without any back and forth.

43 Warm fresh bread.

44 When you like your neighbours.

45 Deep conversations with strangers.

46 Days where you're productive and realise how much you've achieved.

47 The feeling on your skin after you've swum in the ocean.

48 Smelling a fragrance or washing powder on someone else and loving it.

49 Ice cream.

50 A good punchline.

51 Duvet days.

52 Using a notebook for the first time.

53 Reading a story to a toddler as they have their bottle after their bath.

54 Sending silly voice notes back and forth with a friend.

55 Not having to iron something.

56 Inhaling a scent that evokes a happy memory.

57 Looking forward to something in the diary.

58 Cake for breakfast.

59 Seeing your friend happy.

60 Comfortable shoes.

61 Happy tears.

62 A blue sky on an autumnal day.

63 Surprise flowers.

64 Warm gooey cookies.

65 The sound of the rain when you fall asleep.

66 When someone says, 'I love you.'

67 Cheering on your friend.

68 The smell of sunscreen.

69 When you look in the mirror and love your outfit.

70 Gifts for no apparent reason.

71 Holding hands with your grandparent.

72 Having milk in the fridge when someone needs it.

73 A hot shower after being outside all day.

74 When flowers start to bloom.

75 Thinking you'll miss a train but you make it.

76 When the item you were planning on buying suddenly goes on sale.

77 Upgrades.

78 Realising everything is going to be OK.

79 Flying over somewhere beautiful and having a window seat.

80 Photos on film.

81 The smell of your favourite home-cooked meal.

82 Bubbles.

83 Sitting down when you've been on your feet all day.

84 Finding a patch of bluebells or daffodils on a country walk.

85 An appointment cancelling, when you didn't want to go to it anyway.

86 When an animal you love comes to greet you.

87 The feeling of the sun on your face.

88 Waking up and suddenly remembering it's your day off.

89 Seconds after you book the holiday and you have that excited feeling.

90 The air just after it rains.

91 Waking up knowing you went out the night before and still cleansed your face before bed.

92 Making someone smile.

93 Finding you have something in common with someone new.

94 When someone holds the door open for you.

95 That first glimpse of the sea.

96 The sound of a baby laughing.

97 Finding something amazing at an antique market.

98 Free entry to museums.

99 A seat on the train.

100 When a queue of people moves quicker than you expected.

THOUGHTS OF THE DAY

- Wednesday is a day for winning – the prize is more joy, more happiness. How can you get your prize?
- Small can be mighty. Never forget about the tiny tweaks you can make to bring more fun and friendship into your day. Never diminish the impact of a smile, a wave or a compliment. Make Wednesday your day to make small connections with strangers until it becomes a daily habit. If it helps, photograph your glimmers on your phone throughout the week, and save them in a folder so you can check back in on them any time.
- You have so many things to be grateful for. Appreciate the people, places and things that make your heart sing. These are the things that are important. Add something to your own joy list every Wednesday. Just look how long this list can get . . .

Thursday

How other people's energy affects our mood (for an hour, for the day or even our whole week) is something not to be overlooked. When people flow at a low vibration, their energy is off! It's as if they're on a completely different page from you. And this is something we're going to dig into on Thursdays. Yes, gang, it's time to distinguish between your Mood Hoovers and your Energy Radiators.

Before we lean into this, it's important to recognise that this isn't about one of our friends or family members going through a rough patch, perhaps going silent or being sullen or a little difficult. The supporting role we play for our loved ones is vital to us being a well-rounded and kind person. If a person close to us needs help, we will naturally be there, even if it sucks the life force out of us for a little while as we battle to build them up again. But you do need to tune into your instinct about some people you surround yourself with long-term, because there might be people who – if you are really honest with yourself – don't need to be with you on your journey. It's not about disliking someone, or having feelings of animosity. This is about a connection changing, evolving or moving in a direction that feels internally uncomfortable, and just not right for you any more. You owe it to yourself to find the people who make your heart and mind burst with warm sunshine.

Who you have in your day-to-day orbit can directly affect your mood, and having a good healthy attitude around you is an integral part of your self-confidence journey. Your time on Earth is precious, so let's make sure it's as positive as it can be ... You may have heard the saying, 'Friends for a reason, friends for a season'. We need to work out if there are people in your circle who aren't supposed to be in your life any more. There's no better time than this Thursday to start working it out.

During my periods of intense personal growth, I realised that there were some people in my life who really didn't match the place that I was taking myself to. As I learned how to respect myself, and learned my worth in terms of what I bring to the table, I started to understand that if the energy I put out wasn't reciprocated, or the friendship felt very one-sided, then I needed to cut ties. I speak in the past tense here, but this also applies to the present and I'm sure to the future. Being in tune with your values, and what does and doesn't sit right with who you are is a powerful, and sometimes painful, lesson.

I started this Thursday tutorial by referring to friendships, as these have been the most significant element when it comes to erasing certain people from my life. However, this can also apply to colleagues and family members, friends of friends, or your neighbours too. Be aware of how others make you feel. Your energy, your inner power, the core of who you are is an entity that you must work on, constantly and consistently, every day, keeping the optimism up. It doesn't just happen.

CHOPPING ONIONS

What if another person is bringing your joy and positivity down? This is where things can get sticky. Fortunately, however, the act of self-love can be likened to peeling off the layers of an onion. Every time we glow deeper, a layer comes off. When we peel an onion what happens? Sometimes we cry, sometimes we wish we hadn't included it in a recipe, and sometimes – if the dish isn't right – it can even make us ill. But the longer that the peeled layer is separated from the onion, the less pungent it becomes. When it is tolerable, we have the opportunity to decide how we are going to prepare it. Am I going to slice it or mash it? How is it going to be best for me to incorporate it? We're left with a pile of bits of onion, large slices and tiny pieces – and it's time to incorporate the onions into the recipe. Spiritual and life-altering work is much like this. We peel back the layers and experience what there is to be experienced.

YOUR VIBE ATTRACTS YOUR TRIBE

How you are, and who you hang out with, has an effect on the overall version of you. I've lost count of how many times someone has tagged me in a post on social media about being human sunshine. I can confidently say – I am human sunshine! I'm here for the good vibes, the vibrating high vibes, the deep-rooted, life-affirming, heart-warming vibes. I'm not here for shallow emptiness. I'm not here for negativity. Nor am I here for manipulative behaviour, or for being with people who only speak badly of others. Gossip bores me. Social status is irrelevant. As is wealth. Conversations around other people's business, while they can bring a source of low-level entertainment, really don't improve my life or existence in any way, shape or form. Nor will they for you.

ENERGY RADIATORS

There are people in this world who vibrate HIGH! The sun shines out of them: when they walk through the door it's like a breath of spring. Hanging out with them is easy: there's no pretence. Cards on the table – what you see is what you get. Their humour matches yours and you feel safe talking about the hard stuff, knowing there won't be judgement or gossip afterwards. I know my true energy radiators because I either don't care what I look like or how clean my house is before we hang out, or, on the flip side, I make an extra-special effort with how I look or what food I serve because they're a joy to get ready for and be with. Before I see my energy radiators, I'm excited because I know how I'll feel afterwards. Can you recognise any in your life?

- Energy radiators fill your happy cup up to the top.
- You can probably count them on your fingers within seconds.
- They're your cheerleaders, your brass band.
- They love you for who you are, and you love them equally in return.

- You're happy to give your energy to them because you know it will be reciprocated.
- Energy radiators may have been in your life for years, or they might be new. It's an energy, not a timeframe, thing.
- They don't have to have a full-time role in your life – they may be your hairdresser, or a client, a friend of a friend or an aunt. The clue is you never dread seeing them.

MOOD HOOVERS

Sadly, there are some people who, at this present time, do not match your energy. While I'm not telling you to cut anyone out of your life, who you circulate with will make a difference to your journey. If you ask yourself how they make you feel on the inside, there's something about them that would make you answer 'Off'. Until the trigger is pulled to instigate a new thought process towards these people in your life, you might just carry on, which in turn affects your progress. Listen to your instinct. Mood hoovers have the unfortunate ability of changing and shifting the vibe of a group, a moment or a workplace. We've all encountered them. Here are the tell-tale signs:

- You dread seeing them.
- You know that after being around them for a few hours your energy will be lower.
- Conversation is only ever about them and their problems ...
- ... or about commenting on others' appearance or social status ...

- ... and negative gossiping – you don't like how they speak about other people or to other people when you're out with them.
- Conversation with them doesn't feel enriching.
- Telling you ways you can change, or 'improve' yourself that feels critical rather than hopeful.
- Permanent pessimism.
- One-upping.
- Consistent lateness or last-minute cancelling.
- You don't introduce them – or regret introducing them – to your energy radiators.

As I learned to love and respect who I was, I tuned into what was happening when I was with various people. That these behaviours I was witnessing from certain people in my life were not what I gave out to my friends. Things weren't matching. So why was I OK with receiving negativity or mood-hoovering energy in return for the joy I was giving out? Why did I tolerate it?

It all comes down to self-respect. I didn't respect or care about myself enough to confidently erase these people from my life. If you're struggling with your inner light, you can't see who's taking it from you. It can feel like the energy doesn't even have the time to build inside you before someone hoovers it up. It's OK to not hang out with people who don't make you feel good. It's OK to distance yourself from people who aren't bringing you joy. Depending on what space you're in, note that this is not selfish behaviour, but a form of self-protection and preservation. While I realise this might be difficult if a mood hoover is a family member, distance can always ultimately be achieved in one way or another. Not everything has to be dealt with in an official extraditing capacity; mood hoovers usually have enough drama of their own without you adding to it.

WHO LIFTS YOU UP?

We need to let toxic energy out and positivity in. Who are the people who lift you, love you, laugh with you and look after your heart? Value them like the diamonds they are. It's time to raise awareness of who is making you feel good, and who is taking your light.

- Take a piece of paper and draw two columns, one titled 'Radiators', the other titled 'Hoovers'.
- Have a think for a few minutes. Be honest with yourself. Add the names that come to mind to each column.
- Once you have your list of radiators, I want you to contact them. I want you to send them a text:

Hey [insert their name]!
   I need to tell you something – I'm currently reading *The Confidence Ritual* (a book that's designed to spark inner confidence and joy). I've just read a chapter on energy radiators – stay with me here! In the book it tells me that there are people in this world who vibrate HIGH! The sun shines out of them, when they walk through the door it's like a breath of spring. Hanging out with them is easy, there's no pretence. I need to champion my energy

radiators so I'm sending you this text! You are my
energy radiator!! I'm so grateful to have you in my
life, you bring me so much joy, THANK YOU!

Can we hang out or catch up soon? XX

Chances are your energy radiator will send you a text
back filled with joy. Positivity put out into the universe!

If they live near, why not make a plan to meet up,
something extra-special for no reason whatsoever. Maybe
a gallery you've always wanted to visit, or a concert, or
a new cafe that just opened. You could tie it together with
another to-do from your ritual and try a new fitness class.
Do something extra-special with these people and see
how it makes you feel. The excitement on the run-up, the
joy afterwards.

Once the plan is made, why not send an invite! You
can either use Paperless Post or even an electronic calen-
dar invite. If that feels a bit much, text them and let them
know how excited you are to see them. Joy needs celebrating and multiplying!

BUILDING BOUNDARIES AND BARRIERS

It will take time to change how you interact with your mood
hoovers. Creating distance isn't a bad thing, and adding
boundaries into your daily life will help strengthen your
feelings towards them. It's OK to say no. Many people think
boundaries are just physical barriers, like a wall or a moat
designed to keep people out. But when it comes to self-care,

boundaries are not physical, but a powerful way of taking care of ourselves. Since creating boundaries in my life, I am less likely to have feelings of disappointment, hurt and anger towards others. Ultimately, if someone is making you feel bad, you have to protect your light, and put the right boundaries in place.

What will you stand for, and what have you had enough of? Boundaries may come in the form of keeping others at a distance and learning how to say no when something doesn't match your standards. Try not to feel too guilty about setting them up and sticking to them. It's part of putting yourself first. Perhaps the time you spend with another person becomes consciously limited from your side, i.e. because you know, deep down, that any more time with them will negatively affect your mood. Boundaries are also about bringing an awareness to what you truly believe in, and value. So, if someone isn't matching that belief, i.e. behaving in a way you very much disagree with, like being rude to a waiter when you meet at a restaurant, is a boundary needed to distance yourself from them?

Those who are more likely to people-please often lack boundaries because it's easier to say 'Yes' than it is to say 'No'. I remember this from working with certain clients in the past – I found saying no harder because I didn't know what my worth was, which meant I didn't have the confidence to create boundaries. But you are worth so much, and you do not deserve to be treated badly by anyone. Protect your peace, babes. Be consistent with your boundaries. You don't need to advertise your new barriers to everyone, you don't need to tell another person you're setting a boundary . . . just quietly and firmly know within yourself what you will and won't tolerate, and stick to it. If that person continues to cross or push your set boundary repeatedly, then perhaps distance is what's needed.

How to say no

Saying no in your private life doesn't require you to give an explanation to anyone, but sometimes it helps soften the blow or give closure. And in work situations, you might need to explain why you want to say no to something if it is viewed by someone as part of your job. I find honesty is often the best policy, which sadly some struggle with. If saying no feels like a lot – don't be ashamed to back it up. Rather than put the blame onto another ('You always make me feel …)', use 'I' sentences instead.

> *No, I can't, I have other commitments at the moment.*
> *No, I am unable to make that work, but what about another time?*
> *I understand that this matters to you, however I am unable to be what you need right now.*

Remember self-care can be like the layers of an onion: gritty, sticky and stingy in the eyes at first – but eventually palatable. Don't waste any more time, energy and money on people and things that you want to say no to. The more you say no to those things, the more you can give to the big, gorgeous, instant and obvious YES things.

Control who you see on your scroll

Creating content on social media is a job and way of life that I did not expect to find, but I really enjoy it! Social media receives such a bad rep in terms of its addictive nature and the type of content we're shown day to day. Truth is, though, you control your scroll. I'd be kidding myself if I didn't think you've been scrolling on social media daily as you carve out your ritual. However, what we've witnessed with physical energy radiators and mood hoovers in the real world, applies to social media accounts too.

- If you feel like you are comparing yourself to a stranger on the internet, unfollow them.
- If you feel like you are comparing yourself to a friend on the internet, mute them (if you're unsure how to do this, ask a friend or research on the social app's webpages).
- Always remember: how a person is online is not how they are in real life. Fact.
- Engage with accounts that *make you feel good*, and your algorithm will respond with similar content.
- By engaging in accounts that *do not make you feel good* you are curating your social media experience into something that's the opposite of what you want it to be.

To me, social media is a shopfront. What happens to shopfronts on the high street? Well, they display the best stock and change frequently, simply to make you want more and keep you spending. That's what social media is – it's a person's or company's shopfront, but it's never the true story. There is always something going on behind the scenes. It's a digital life curated to engage you during your time on the apps. I'll never tell you not to scroll on social media – I love that we are exposed to so much of humanity and there is such a freedom in being on the apps. Voices are amplified! However, you control the decks. You have the power to curate and manipulate your algorithm as you so wish. And you must!

How someone else chooses to live their life on their social media account is their business. How you choose to engage and who you follow is your choice, and your choice alone. For example, I do not follow any of the Kardashians on Instagram, not because I don't like them, but because I don't like the content that they put out – it doesn't align with my values and what I want my scroll to look like. And I have muted many peers on social media, not because I don't like them personally, but because their content does not align with how I want to feel. You control the scroll, babes. Always.

THOUGHTS OF THE DAY

- Remember you are now actively being aware of who is bringing you joy, and who is taking your joy. Revisit your friends and family list regularly to make sure you're sticking with – and valuing – the radiators, the sunshine bringers. This is where you begin to curate who you circulate with – it's not indulgent, it's important.

- As this ritual is YOUR ritual, and this is your new way of life, it doesn't need to be openly discussed with other people (unless you want it to be). If you are choosing to consciously curate who you give your energy to and receive it from – this is your business. It doesn't need yelling through a megaphone.

- Setting boundaries is one of the healthiest things you can do for yourself. Thursday can work as a reminder that – yes – walking away from friendships or family members is very hard, so hard you might think it's impossible . . . but you must be a friend to yourself first. Recommit to this every week.

- Your social circle, your social media . . . you are the curator of it all. Feel free to cut. Each Thursday have a little self-edit of who is taking up your time.

- Your energy is precious cargo. Treat it, and yourself, with respect – you're absolutely worth it!

Friday

Friday is for the Wardrobe Warrior. Although I don't work in fashion or styling, I have some advice to share. Clothes and how we present ourselves, our overall outward look, play a huge part in how we reach peak glow status. Contrary to popular opinion, however, I don't believe that the clothes make a full outfit. Clothes don't glow, they don't beam confidence, they don't have an energy to them – that's your job!

As I began incorporating *The Confidence Ritual* into my life, I naturally began to dress differently. Rather than a sea of black, or play-it-safe options, I started to experiment with colour and shapes, and learned to fine-tune my personal styling. This linked to what was on- or off-brand for me, which made it easier and smarter when shopping. Rather than a wardrobe filled with pieces that I liked that didn't quite sit together, or what felt like a dozen of the same thing (black skinny jeans), I consciously curated my wardrobe so that every time I got dressed it became joyful.

How we navigate our wardrobe and choose what to wear – or what not to wear – is up to us. Clothes have a big role in the confidence journey, and so now we activate your inner wardrobe warrior! Which items of our clothing make us feel great, strong and powerful? Why do they make us feel great, what's so special about them? The colour? The fabric? The cut? Think about what's in your wardrobe that sparks dopamine, because dopamine dressing is where we're headed . . .

In the darkest depths of my body dysmorphia, I placed so much of my worth on the letter or number denoting my clothes size. As I dieted, I became fixated on being able to get into a smaller size. Equally, as I put weight back on and my body changed again, I would torture myself by comparing the varying clothes sizes, often resulting in tears and self-shame. Using clothes labels as a form of self-valuing has to stop. I've managed it, and I want to share how. Let's unpack your wardrobe – let's start on Friday in time for your weekend plans.

SIZE MEANS NOTHING

I had a knitwear brand for a short period of time, until drastic economic shifts and a surge in production costs meant the brand simply couldn't survive. During the time when we manufactured the garments, it was totally up to us as brand founders to decide how we saw our garments fitting; how wide and long would a 'small' be v. a 'large', for example. Sure, there were 'industry standards' as a guideline, but these were pretty flexible. When you mix that insider knowledge with the fact that many retailers are based in different countries, where people come in all manner of shapes and sizes, you have a completely unregulated, guesstimate of garment-size-scape. What is a small to one person is a medium to another.

A person who thinks they are a size 10 might fit a 12 in one style, but an 8 in another. There is no guide, no rule, no real meaning to any of it.

If you're like I used to be, whereby the size of the garment means a huge deal to you – babe, I get it, but please trust me when I say there is another way of shopping. You can still use your preferred size as your trusty guide, but if something waivers either side of that number, you can navigate that moment with optimism, believe me! Tears in the fitting room are no laughing matter; I have lost count of how many times I have cried in there. The wrong size, too tight, snooty shop assistants, pulling my body apart in the mirror. It's the worst! It can ruin a perfectly good day!

How we shop and wear clothes is something I really want to tackle head-on, because I remember clearly how clothes size once ruled my life. Fashion wasn't fun, it was torture … but I didn't need to drop a dress size. My body was never the problem: the way I viewed the situation was.

Whereas I used to deem my worth according to the number in the back of a pair of trousers, now I just see a pair of trousers, nothing more, nothing less. If they fit, great, if not OK – let's go up a size. To some this might sound simple; to others, it might mean a whole lot of mental discomfort. Either way, remember that nobody sees that number. If it's causing that much mental strain, cut the label out the moment you get the clothing home. Life is just too short to place your worth on an unregulated size label in the back of a garment.

NAMING YOUR STYLE

How I felt within my body ultimately had a knock-on effect on how I dressed and the clothes I chose to wear. Living a life as a backstage beauty expert ultimately meant that for the majority of my twenties I wore all black. When I launched my own product line I suddenly went from backstage to front of house and did not know how to dress! A sucker for fast fashion, I bought bright colours, loud prints and poorly made garments. I had no idea what I was doing. My wardrobe was messy – there was no theme, which meant that my clothes didn't align with one another, and pieces weren't interchangeable. It wasn't a good use of my money. Quick hits with no longevity.

A tip I picked up from a fashion stylist I worked with on a shoot once was to theme my wardrobe – creating key words I could go to when shopping or when organising pieces I already owned. I'd love you to think about doing this too. Spend a few minutes thinking about what makes you feel happy, confident and what you'd love as your signature style, then head to your wardrobe. If an item fits your theme, keep it. If not, don't put in back in there.

So how do you set your style?

- Pinterest can be a very useful place to start looking for ideas.
- Try consciously noticing who you look at when walking down the street or flicking through a magazine or scrolling on social media. Who is turning your head, and why? I'm not referring to any degree of negative comparison here – this is strictly for

inspiration. Who's got something you want, and what is it?!

- I began by researching what I wanted my wardrobe to look and feel like: did I want to be polished or relaxed?
- When I thought about who I was on the inside, it helped me carve out how I wanted to present myself on the outside. What messages or energy do you want to put out to the world, and what look would help?
- Think about what you are spending your hard-earned cash on! Are you going to wear this again and again? Is it timeless or is it a trend?

I hate feeling uncomfortable, and cannot understand the point of wearing something that doesn't *feel good*. It's like wearing an itchy school blazer! Get it off! That simple mindset shift in turn helped me when I was shopping. I'd ask myself, am I comfortable? Is this making me feel relaxed?

If the answer was no, I simply wouldn't buy it (this might seem obvious to some of you but to others, like my past self, forcing my body into clothes that weren't right for my shape was the norm!). The feeling of comfort then helped me decide what fabrics I wanted to wear. If something wasn't feeling good on my skin, then why would I wear it?

If you're not familiar with wardrobe words, I've listed some below. Theming your wardrobe then helps when you shop. You can pick up a garment and ask yourself if this fits with your theme; this not only makes the shopping experience a whole lot easier, but also helps to make your wardrobe interchangeable. Spend time sitting and looking at what and who comes up in your search engines when you input these words. The words I use for my style are timeless, celestial and Americana. While we're predominately referring to clothing here, this will also weave its way into your beauty look and how you choose to dress your skin and style your hair.

Romantic
Boho
Sleek Chic
Tailored
Rocker
Relaxed / Casual
Glam
Beachy
Minimalist
Androgynous
Sexy
Preppy
Avant-garde
Urban
Elegant
Athletic
Corporate
Western/Americana
Celestial/Whimsical
Sixties
Seventies
Eighties
Nineties
Y2K

YOU GOT THE LOOK

Set a scene – put some of your favourite music on, light a scented candle (even light the one you've been saving for a special occasion!), make your favourite drink and fall down the style rabbit hole. Set aside an hour if you can, and really lean into your research. Don't worry about what your wardrobe or style looks like now: think about where and who you want to be. Don't think about the shape of your body or the colour of your hair – this has nothing to do with that. This is simply about what you are drawn to. The process is not indulgent, this is a form of inner investment to future you. This research is sourcing inspiration that lights you up. You can of course use more than three words to define your wardrobe, but be warned: the more you have the harder it can be to shop and piece outfits together.

WHAT'S IN THE WARDROBE?

If you never bought another item of clothing, would you be happy with what you have in your wardrobe? Have you curated your style so that when you shop for a new item, you know it will work with clothes you already own, rather than panic-buy one-off, trend-driven and potentially unsuitable piece?

Open up your wardrobe and what do you see? Are your clothes neatly organised? Do you sort by colour? Or is it a rambling set of chaos? Perhaps you have matching hangers, or maybe you have an assortment of dry cleaners' hangers? Either way, how you have your wardrobe sorted (or not) is none of my business, that's your space. For the record mine's a combination of organised chaos meets strict system. It's a beast of its own, if you will! Now I want you to answer these questions so you can dissect what's in there.

Has everything been worn?
Are there items in there still with tags on?
Do you wear some items on repeat?
Do you avoid wearing other items because they're
  uncomfortable?
Are other items collecting dust and taking up space?
Are you saving anything for best?
Are you holding on-to items because you might one day fit
  back into them?

I found that having items in my wardrobe that I wanted so badly to fit back into when I lost weight made the getting-ready process painful. Every day as I opened my wardrobe, I was reminded of the person I used to be. I had no idea that I was self-sabotaging my chances at gaining more confidence, letting those items haunt me and remind me of my past self, a version of me that was never coming back.

I was holding on to a pair of trousers that, looking back, I have no idea how they ever fitted me. When I look at photos of me wearing them, I look like a different person, lost and unhappy. I held onto them, starved myself again and got back into them once more, only to be equally as unhappy as I was the time before. It took me years to get rid of them, but once

I did, giving them to my younger female cousin, the release I felt became a focus for me. How the physical act of removing something from my wardrobe was almost like shaking off a past version of me. I was letting go and breaking free. This was a tipping point: I started looking at my wardrobe with a more logical and critical eye. While clothes won't make you feel body confident on the inside, they are still a true cloak of our subconscious. Think about this:

Are you wearing your clothes to feel good or look thin?
Are you dressing to seek someone else's approval or are you going for comfort?
Perhaps you feel like your wardrobe could also do with a glow up or even a curation?
Are we dressing for how we feel or simply what we think we should be wearing?

WARDROBE WARRIORS

I want you to be truly honest with yourself because this is a huge part of the glow up journey and you're going to have to put up a good fight to get where you need to be. Be brave.

- Open up your drawers and cupboards, and answer these questions.

What is in your wardrobe that you're holding on to?
What pieces are in there that you know, deep down, have had their moment?

What isn't coming back round again?

When you revisit the three words you've chosen to describe your wardrobe, which items make the cut, and which don't?

- Once you've thought about this, clear out what is no longer working. This might be one piece, it might be half a dozen, you might fill four bin liners. Go to your wardrobe and drawers and get these items out. Enough is enough: they once brought you joy but now don't serve your purpose any more. As Italian tenor Andrea Bocelli says – it's time to say goodbye! Perhaps the fabric reminds you of a time you want to forget, or maybe when you try something on and look at yourself in the mirror, you simply feel off. That's your cue. If it's not feeling right on the inside, why are we doing it on the outside?

- Time to put on a playlist and treat this as an act of self-love. This is you, unpacking a part of your life and wishing it well. This is you, making space for newness to come in.

- As you choose the pieces, thank them for the joy they brought you. Make this process ritualistic. Speak to the higher being if necessary. Say out loud 'Thank you!' but don't sit and dwell on the memories; a photo can do just the same. Be swift with the assassination.

- What you do with these pieces is entirely up to you – you might wish to donate them to a charity, or gift them to a family member or friend. Perhaps you

want to sell them? If you do my advice is not to
focus on price; just focus on the fact they're going
to another person who'll give them a whole new
life.

- If they can be altered in any way, go for it, give them
  a whole new lease of life! Maybe you want to repurpose them as tea towels or napkins, you do you!
- Whatever you choose to keep or clear out remember,
  make your wardrobe work for you.

FOR THE WEEK AHEAD

What is in your wardrobe that could be worn this week? I
want you to pull out one or two pieces and hang them
somewhere in your eyeline, so they have to be worn this
week. And not just clothes – it could be shoes, activewear,
jewellery, a handbag, even a hat! If you've spent money on an
item and it's not being worn – what's going on? If you work
in an environment that dictates your wardrobe professionally,
perhaps there's casual Friday – could this be the day you
bring out something you haven't worn in ages? Is there
something you're going to on Friday evening that could be
the perfect scenario for an old favourite to make an
appearance? Maybe you're spending your Friday night in – is
this where you dive deep and allow yourself the time to
research your style?

We can fall into the habit of wearing the same thing every
week, and when it comes to getting dressed up, we choose
our regular clothes but add a lipstick or an earring. Can we go

that bit further for ourselves? Can we push to step into a version of ourselves we truly want to be?

Many of the weekly tasks talked about in Part Two can interlink with one another, so please don't feel overwhelmed by every shift that's happening – you can completely go at your own pace. Take note of what comes out of your wardrobe this week. As you make plans to bring joy through the week, think about wearing these items to elevate the occasion even more. Life is too short and special to save anything for best. Believe me, your day-to-day is worthy of best!

THOUGHTS OF THE DAY

- As your wardrobe begins to take shape, the items that make you feel bad will disappear and you'll be left with a wardrobe that sparks joy and is quicker and easier to navigate.
- Sorting out your style might feel like an overwhelming task at first, but the wardrobe workload will diminish quickly because the clear-out will help cultivate your wardrobe and get it organised.
- Whenever you need to pack a bag for a trip – be it work, pleasure, overseas vacation or weekend away with the girls – pack items in your case that you haven't worn or you're saving for best. This then gives the items no choice but to go into rotation. Nothing should be saved for a rainy day. You don't know what weather is in the forecast.
- Do this for you. I want everything you wear to make you feel happy, comfortable and confident. Dopamine dressing is your new way of life!

Saturday

On Saturdays, we get to consciously tune into everything we've learned or implemented throughout the week so far; to dig a little deeper and embed the practical changes we need to make, harnessing everything in our power to make ourselves glow from the inside out – and this includes focusing on the spiritual side of things.

COULD IT BE MAGIC?

Manifesting is not a new phenomenon. Manifesting is prayer, repackaged. For centuries humans have offered themselves to a higher purpose, made offerings and sacrifice, and shone their hope upwards, PRAYING for change to come. And at times, change arrived. I've manifested and believed in the law of attraction since I skimmed through Rhonda Byrne's *The Secret* when I was eighteen years old; a self-help book with messages that felt so obvious to me, I think I actually said, 'Well, duh!' as I threw it onto my bed. If you haven't read it, it's a brilliant explanation of how the law of attraction works, tuning into what you truly desire in life and being aware of when the right doors open. I believe manifesting is closely linked to this. As you become aware of what you want, you consciously make a decision to list out things that you desire in your life.

I may have always manifested, but I have also always believed there is an element of knuckling down to getting the job done. Manifesting will only take you so far. There, I said it. We can't just dream about something; we need to put some work in. I see it as linking the daydreamer to the grafter. Focusing on what you really want and setting goals for where you want to go, and then actually doing the work to get yourself there. I do believe that my husband, my career, our gorgeous house – even the colour and breed of our dog – are all partly down to manifesting. I believe manifesting *helped* build the dream life I am in now. When I was working backstage, I always had in my head a clear vision of what I wanted to achieve – I held an inner hope that the path I had chosen would pay off, and it did.

I'm fortunate to have been spiritually tuned in my whole life. I'm not afraid of dying, for example, because I'm pretty certain I'll be coming back round, yet again. My parents tell me I used to speak to spirits in my bedroom, and I can tell you if I think a house is haunted or not within half an hour of being inside. It's a feeling. My atheist medic brother would wholeheartedly disagree, because he has a science brain, beautifully curated by fact. The same applies to many of the medics I have met: their job has taught them to disconnect emotion from death or illness. Life is linear.

However, science and spirituality came from the same place – the stars. Both astrology and astronomy are studies of the stars. Astronomy helps us to understand our universe, and astrology seeks to help us understand ourselves within it.

Joe Marcin, science journalist and author of *Human Cosmos*, stated recently on a podcast: '... right from prehistoric times, people were really interested in the sky, it was part of their everyday life. And that's because what was happening in the sky really was crucial for what was happening on earth ... throughout the night, the stars are turning around in the sky, they're giving you a sub-sense of time.' Whether you look to the stars and see planets, atoms and physics, or whether you see and feel a higher being – you're looking up and feeling something. The stars might be pointing your life in a direction you either do or don't accept or believe in. The stars might give you feelings of hope. You may feel both. What seems clear to one person might seem murky to another, and there is no right or wrong answer. While I'm a huge believer in the power of manifesting, I truly believe the power of the deepest manifest comes to you when everything else runs in unison. Life needs to be in a state of flow for abundance to flourish.

What do I mean by this? Well, as you change up your week, you've actively chosen to bring a sense of awareness and purpose into your existence. As you build in all the different aspects, on rotation, week on week, your life begins to shift and things will tend to feel that bit easier – life starts to flow. Routine becomes ritual. As this shift begins, and you then add extras like manifesting, getting what you desire becomes easier because you're already in a place of high-vibing positive energy. There's a lack of pessimism because you've tackled the things that drain your energy. Perhaps you no longer fear failure, because you can recognise failure isn't a negative thing. You're choosing to surround yourself with energy frequencies that match your own, and you have your own inner light in clear focus. You're now focusing on *you*.

Manifesting is a powerful tool in creating inner guidelines. It helps set clear aims, and identifies your truest desires, which in turn makes it easier to visualise what you want. Setting about manifesting requires realism: hope, of course, has to be ignited, but so does a framework that puts your inner state of joy at the front of your existence. I love manifesting, but to me manifesting is simply a spoke in the umbrella of ritual. It's OK creating a vision board but unless your practice is backed up by theory and doing the actual work, it's unlikely your vision board will truly take off.

Vision boards and manifesting do help you shape up a desired visualisation for where you see yourself being in the future – it's almost like putting your desires as co-ordinates into a sat nav. The destination is programmed, the route is set – but, honey, you have to drive. If you say it over and over enough (just like ancient prayer), subconsciously you'll begin putting the wheels in motion and things will start to happen – whether you believe it's the universe or determination, or a combination of both. Perhaps you're manifesting love, or peace, or a new job, or maybe you're being really specific and manifesting a holiday far away! Who knows what's on your manifesting wish list? My point is – it's yours.

DREAMS DO COME TRUE –
WITH DETERMINATION

When my husband and I lived in London, we spent many weekends away in the countryside, escaping from the city. One day, when we were relaxing in a pub beer garden, I said,

'We should create a vision cloud together.' My husband, an atheist, rolled his eyes. 'C'mon, it'll be fun!' I said. While he got another round in, I ran to our holiday cottage and fetched a pen and paper.

In the middle I wrote our names and drew a cloud shape around them. From there I mind-mapped what was in our heads and where we saw our life going. We could write ANYTHING we wanted – whatever was in our head, or in our dreams. One by one our dreams appeared on that piece of paper.

A house!
A detached house!
A house with a palm tree!
A dog! A dog that looks like a deer! A calm, gentle dog that we rescued!
The sea, we're near the sea!
Both financially stable.
An hour from the city.
Another animal, not sure what, but another animal.
Kids!

We filled the page and had fun doing it. It was gorgeous to read my husband's wishes. The point is, they were all out in the open and down on the page. We could visualise our life together. We put the pad away and life carried on for a few more years. . . . And then, in 2020, we left London and moved into a renovation project. Our life sat in boxes as we slowly worked our way around the house, changing and modifying it to what we wanted it to be. Most of our belongings stayed in those boxes until we'd finished the major work.

In the year we got married, we unpacked a box that contained the visualised mind-map we'd created in that beer garden and I stood staring at it in disbelief. There I was in our detached house, with a palm tree in the garden and a rescue dog that looked like a deer sitting calmly and quietly next to me. We were in the Kentish countryside, fifteen minutes from the sea, and an hour from London. We were both financially stable. There are still some things missing as I write this book, but I am certain they will come to us. We will make sure they come to us.

Whether you believe that this is manifesting, or that it's simply a to-do checklist, doesn't matter – it happened before my very eyes. What I desired came to me, with every specification met. Now, every January, I host workshops on how to set your goals for the year ahead. At the start of every year, I visualise what I truly want in the year, and things happen! This book deal was one of them! I manifested this book deal . . . alongside the help of my literary agent, publisher, social media following, a carefully crafted pitch and of course, physically writing it, I have become a published author! You can do anything you put your mind to. Whether that's down to determination or magic – or most likely, I believe, a combination of the two – you have the power to visualise and turn aspirations into reality.

NEGATIVE MANIFESTING

Be warned! While we hear much about the true magic of manifestation, little is spoken of *negative* manifesting. It's important to address that there can also be darker forces at play when manifesting is not done correctly. Negative manifesting is something we're usually unaware of doing. It's when the inner pessimist comes to the surface, or we allow ourselves to listen to bullies or gossips, or to that negative voice that sometimes resides within us when we've lost our glow.

I can recall talking to my therapist about someone I was really struggling with at that time in my life, and they replied, 'Pessimism is a form of protection.' Everything became clear for me at that moment. Pessimism *is* a total form of protection. We push our negative thoughts forward to deflect showing what we truly want or to disguise our fear of failing. Pessimism is a deflection of insecurity. It conceals trauma. Pessimism blocks high vibrational optimistic rays. It's the mud that you get stuck in. When pessimism is at play, we run the risk of manifesting things we truly do *not* want or desire.

If you repeatedly tell yourself you hate your body, then that will be your reality. You will spend the rest of your life hating your body. If you tell yourself you won't get that promotion, or you won't find love, or perhaps you won't achieve the life you've always wanted, then that will be your reality. Being honest with yourself about what you truly desire, and allowing yourself to open up with vulnerability and honesty, will help raise your vibrations. Pessimism will do nothing but deflect the goodness from shining in.

I see it so often: individuals who have *the dream life* – the house, the car, the babies, the holidays, all the boxes ticked in terms of what we 'should' have – yet they're unhappy. Deep down, you can see the light is trying so hard to glimmer but is dulled with pessimism and negative manifesting. There's a desire for even more materialism and perfectionism, even fame, and a lack of inner peace and vibrational flow. I've encountered many individuals who, from the outside, appear successful and who are extremely wealthy and have everything the mind could desire ... but their hearts lie empty. They're not happy. The more you put the negative and toxic out, the more the universe will believe it's what you truly want.

Recognising negative manifesting and putting a stop to it, will help raise your inner optimist and in turn your phoenix. Never forget that your physical life doesn't have to change, just your viewpoint. Be careful how and what you manifest!

CREATE YOUR PERSONAL MANIFESTATION CLOUD

You can manifest on whatever day of the week you want, but to me there is no better day than Saturday, after you've successfully completed a week of implementing and upkeeping your new rituals. With the wheels already in motion, let's now visualise.

- Sitting with the knowledge and feeling of achievement from everything you've completed and actioned within the last week, clear a calm space to begin your visualisation. If you have a busy, noisy household, Saturday might not be the easiest day to manifest, but if there's an hour, or even half an hour, to focus, prioritise this.
- Take a piece of paper and write your name in the middle, draw a cloud shape around it and slowly begin adding arrows, pointing away from the cloud.
- What do you want in life? If you close your eyes and visualise the life you've always dreamed of, what's

there? Write down these things at the end of each arrow.

- Think of your senses – what can you see, smell, hear, feel? Add these wants and wishes to the end of the arrows, too.
- Remember: there is no 'wrong' manifestation cloud – it's exactly as you wish it to be.
- If you're feeling crafty, then really go for it – cut out pictures, stick them on the board!
- After I've have written down my desires, I love to sit on Pinterest and deep dive, creating a digital version of my manifestation cloud.
- Now you begin to see everything you truly desire.

I like to include all areas of my life, but I'm not expecting the universe to bring me everything at once. I have accepted that the universe knows when I'm ready, and when I'm not.

Take breaks if you can, keep staring at the page and allow other desires to surface. Categorise them if you like: career, where you live, who's with you, financial status – get it all down.

This might not be your first time reading *The Confidence Ritual*. If you're re-reading, you may wish to check back in on the previous manifestation cloud and ask yourself if anything came to light?

YOUR ROAD MAP

Your manifestation cloud is there to show you everything you truly desire deep down, but I believe – unlike many of the wellness industry voices out there offering their advice – manifesting will only take you so far. So how do we turn our dreams into reality? How do we get anywhere on the best route? We need a road map! The road map is how you're going to create and bring in what you desire.

> *Who do you know who might be able to open the doors you*
> *want?*
> *What actions do you need to take to turn your manifestation*
> *cloud from thoughts to physical matter?*

Let's get practical. Take a sheet of A3 paper and turn it on its side in landscape orientation. In the middle of the left-hand side write *I Am Here*, with today's date underneath. On the other side write *I Am Here*, with a date you will be working towards. It could be in a year's time, it could be six months, it could be five years. Whatever it is, set a goal. Join the two versions of you up with an arrow pointing to the right-hand side and think about:

> *How are you going to get there?*
> *What needs weeding out?*
> *What needs bringing in?*
> *Who can help you?*

In the place where you want to be, write down how you feel. Be specific about everything you want to achieve, and have in your power the future version of you. If your aim is to feel better, or more confident – how are you consciously going to achieve that? By now you've identified your energy radiators; you might have a new hobby pending or you may be about to try a new workout class. Write these things on your road map so that you can clearly visualise how you're going to get to the mental place you desire.

I strive to be living in a constant state of mental peace, where creativity flows, and I am free of energies that drain my joy. I have curated a space where I can float in a state of wholesome euphoria. It didn't just happen; I had to put my wishes at the forefront and begin implementing change, and the same might be true for you. Write it all down and believe in your power that change will come.

On Saturdays we take a mental check-in of where we've come from and where we're going. If this is the first time you've created your manifestation cloud and road map, enjoy the process and the time it takes to put together. If this is your second or third week working through The Confidence Ritual, check back in on your cloud, look at your road map and consciously ignite or reignite the changes. Perhaps on this Saturday you're on the way to completing some of your checklists from your ritual? Are you clearing out the wardrobe? Have you just exercised with someone who brings you joy? Have you made plans to be in nature? Maybe you're going out of your comfort zone, attending an event you couldn't have seen yourself at a year ago, wearing an item of clothing that you know brings you comfort and confidence and reflects who you are on the inside? I hope you are spending some time doing something solely for you.

THOUGHTS OF THE DAY

- It's Saturday; it's happening, you're doing it. Take a moment to be present with your hopes and – whether you believe that science or spirituality is guiding you there – appreciate how your ship of inner confidence is turning.

- As *The Confidence Ritual* starts to move into its own flow in your life, Saturday can become a day where you check back in on your manifestation cloud and road map. It's good to see what's been achieved and what it feels like is in motion.

- Saturday then becomes a day that frees itself up for you to catch up on other repetitive rituals from the week. Can you add in another workout? Can you see another friend? Maybe you can nature bathe while spending time with your family, like a true high-vibin' multitasker. Perhaps you now have a free hour for naked dancing in your bedroom! Whatever healthy, happy thing it is, never forget to go for it, babes!

The Confidence Ritual Checklist

This might feel like a lot to take in, but I know YOU have the power to change YOUR life. There is a better, healthier way of thinking, feeling and being. I know you can do this!

This book's advice and exercises will become your ritual; your daily, weekly, monthly practice to keep you on track – keeping your vibrations high and living life as the best version of you. Slowly but surely, *The Confidence Ritual* will help you navigate low self-esteem and negative body image by practising self-love on repeat.

Let's recap and make a plan!

SUNDAY

- Soft Sundays are where it's at – go easy and prep for the week ahead.
- Mentally offload anything that's holding you back and get rid of it in the Fuck It Bucket. Journal if you feel like it.
- Make your plan and book onto a fitness class or commit to doing one piece of movement or exercise

this week. If this feels like a struggle, re-read the section on fitness before you do it (it's on page 113).

- If you're into it, have a Spa Sunday. You don't have to spend ages in the bathroom, but I always find a mask and a lick of self-tan on my face helps me combat negativity on Mondays.

MONDAY

- We're reframing Monday; she's had a bad rep in the past and we're not treating her with grunts and groans any more! Monday is going to become your new favourite day!
- Weighing scales OUT – diet does not start on Monday.
- If you don't hit the snooze button for one day in your entire week, make it Monday. Set your alarm for the time you truly wish to wake up.
- Avoid doom scrolling – remember this is going to affect your day negatively – and keep your mind clear.
- Hydrate, because present self looks after future self. If you're feeling bloated today this will help reduce tomorrow's bloat.
- Take thirty minutes outside – nature bathe, baby! Whether it's having your morning drink outside, or taking a walk on your lunch break, try to find some green and take it in!

TUESDAY

- The day begins with writing down five things you're grateful for, in particular towards your body. Focus on all the goodness you already have in place and all that your body does for you!

- Take time to be consciously naked. Spend a few extra minutes being naked and taking in your body as you look at yourself in the mirror.
- Be aware of how you talk about your body to others, and how others in turn talk about their body to you. Consciously activate a chat filter where you recognise it's a choice to engage in conversations around negative body image, and that you're no longer vibing at that frequency. Say NO to negativity.

WEDNESDAY

- While Wednesday may feel like the hump in the middle of the working week, it can be a powerful place to focus on feeding and fuelling your inner joy.
- If there is a sense of loneliness in your life, or perhaps you feel your vibrations are low, let's actively raise them by focusing on your present. Who can you wave to? A local shopkeeper, your dry cleaner, a fellow dog walker, or someone where you buy your coffee or lunch close to where you work? Wednesday is for saying, 'Hi!'
- On Wednesday perhaps you can think about what your glimmers (those small pockets of joy in your week) would be. If it's a physical thing, don't forget to take a photo and save it in an album in your phone.
- Wednesday is for finding your happy – that's the soul and sole purpose of it. Is it calling a good friend and making plans? Is it kitchen dancing to your favourite

radio show? Maybe it's eating a favourite meal? Whatever you choose to do to make yourself feel happier, acknowledge that you are consciously manipulating your day to bring yourself more joy. You're beginning to conjure your inner power.

THURSDAY

- Today we're bringing awareness to our energy radiators and mood hoovers. Who is giving us light, and who is taking it?
- While this might feel like a tough task at first, it's never easy consciously distancing ourselves from people who don't make us feel good – and it doesn't all have to be done at once.
- Carving out boundaries is something that takes time, and the more you dive deeper into creating your ritual, the more your inner voice and intuition will rise up. It will become easier to tune into your inner vibrations because every other aspect of this ritual aims to raise them!
- The people who make you feel good are the ones worth giving your energy to. When you begin distancing yourself from your mood hoovers the change won't happen overnight. I recommend tuning into how you feel pre- and post meet-up and bring a level of awareness into your social interactions. More time with your radiators, less time with your hoovers.
- If you feel lower after hanging out with someone, make a note of it. It might be a one-off – your instinct

will tell you if it is or isn't. If this is consistently happening, you'll know deep down if it's time to focus more on the radiators than the hoovers.

- Remember to send a text (or find another way to reach out) to your energy radiators!
- Think about and curate who you follow on social media – remember – you control the scroll.

FRIDAY

- It's time to channel your inner wardrobe warrior! Today you are going to wear something that makes you feel great. You're going to dress for your dopamine and WEAR YOUR WARDROBE!
- If you work from home, you have no excuse. There's no dress code – and even if you're doing video calls, you can still wear your favourite skirt or trousers! Heck, it could even be a beloved pair of socks!
- Equally, if something is sitting in your wardrobe unworn, it's time to wheel it out. You didn't buy it to hang in your wardrobe, so let's consciously curate our outfit with inner joy.
- Jewellery, hair clips, bags – you name it, let's be wearing it. Even a different necklace, or a ring you've forgotten you had, will help give you a feeling of freshness.
- If you have a corporate role that dictates what you wear to work, maybe you bought something for the office that you haven't really worn enough? Perhaps you're in a place of wardrobe repetition? Is there an item in your wardrobe that needs to be brought into rotation?

- Equally, if you like, this day can be moved to another day in the week (this is your ritual, remember!). Perhaps you have something coming up at the weekend where you want to wear something special? Is there something in the wardrobe that needs dusting off and parading?
- Rather than scrolling nonsense on social media, can you set that time aside to think and research your wardrobe themes? Pinterest is a great place to fall down style rabbit holes. Remember to go with what you feel called to. Can you bring styling inspiration to yourself? If you like it, then, honey, wear it!

SATURDAY

- It's time for you to create (or revisit) your manifestation cloud and road map. Set aside time in your day to hone in on what you want in life – what do you see yourself achieving?
- Once this is out and set, we can check back in on where we're at, and see if we can begin to cross things off the list. Remember: some things happen fast, others take time, and that's OK. Having a spiritual strategy isn't a bad thing: lean in and let it flow!
- Saturday is also a day where we can catch up on our ritual and anything we might have missed in the week. While I love the idea of everything being completed on the day I've set for it, you're in control of your own life. Your working week and your structure will no doubt differ from mine, so build this ritual around YOU.

Epilogue

Recognising that you wish to improve and implement change isn't easy! Go You! As you begin to realign your world, allow this ritualistic way of being to evolve naturally and take its shape and form around you. Go easy with yourself during the process. It's a lot to take on board, and if you miss a day that's OK – just pick it back up the following day. The most important thing is that you keep your ritual flowing.

Creating new and healthy habits for both mind and body won't fall into place overnight – the good stuff takes time, so why rush something that's so rewarding? Becoming aware of your actions, your inner power, who you spend your time with – it's a lot to take on board! If it feels like it's ever getting too much, remember to journal or nature bathe – or both – because these two things will help calm and relax you, and get you back in balance. You are totally in control at all times – that's the beauty of creating this change – but sometimes we need to be reminded of that.

GO WITH THE GLOW

If it helps, why not copy out the Ritual Bingo card below? This way you have something physical pinned up somewhere obvious (the fridge, your desk at work or your bathroom mirror) to check in on and cross off.

- Book an exercise class.
- Complete an exercise class.
- Contact an energy radiator.
- Hang out with my energy radiator.
- Identify an activity that makes me feel good.
- Do said activity that makes me feel good.
- Find my style words.
- Create a playlist of my favourite mood-boosting songs.
- Add photos of small moments of joy to a glimmer photo album on my phone.
- Find one piece of clothing or an accessory (old or new) that makes me feel good.
- Wear that piece of clothing or accessory!
- Unfollow accounts that do not make me feel good.
- Enjoy an at-home spa Sunday.
- Write a gratitude list about my body.
- Focus on my body gratitude list when I look in the mirror.
- Create a manifestation cloud.
- Create a road map.
- Nature bathe.

As you'll have noted throughout the book, I refer to my life before *The Confidence Ritual* as my past life. Perhaps you will too, because eventually it does feel like that. Maybe *The Confidence Ritual* has brought up feelings from the past for you, or identified problems you have in your present? Keep saying aloud, 'This is part of my journey' – because it is!

Curate moments in your life that you are fully aware of, and recognise the joyful benefits they bring. Being aware of how these moments will affect your future is smart spiritual living! Lean. In. Honey! Those who neglect the journey bypass the shift to becoming the person they really desire to be! Hits deep, doesn't it?

Sharing with you the moments in my life that have led me to this place, teaching you the art of the inner glow up, well . . . the honour is all mine. I must express intense gratitude to you for trusting in my guidance and absorbing the way of life that saved me from a dark path and gave me the high-vibing life I live now. It worked for me, and I know it can work for you too.

Doing the work isn't always easy; sometimes it's gritty, and the easiest thing to do would be to give up. But when you're close to throwing in the towel, that is the moment you say no to yourself, and you get back on the self-love train – that's where the growth happens. When you want to give up, but you choose to keep going – that's strength.

Let it get gritty. Choose the hard path if you have to, work on your friendship circle and syphon off the people, places and things that don't make you feel good. With each shift you implement in your life, there may be tears, an uncomfortable feeling, or pain. Think of the onion, those layers coming off, one by one! The moments that hurt in the past are in the past – I don't have a time machine, and neither do you, so don't dwell on them. Pain brings healing, which in turn creates strength. Babes, use it all to fire up what's really inside you. The comments someone said to you, the things you're holding on to . . . Just by reading this book, you've activated your senses and you've pulled the lever to becoming a happier version of you. Your vibrations are rising, like the beautiful phoenix you are! Commit to yourself.

One last warning: *The Confidence Ritual* is yours now; you are changing YOUR life, getting out there and LIVING IT. Not everyone is going to have your back while you embark on this journey, and this new high-vibing version of you may cause unsettlement in others. As you focus your energy inward, others might struggle to understand what's happening. That's their stuff. You cannot control how other people respond to the higher version of you. As you dig deeper to unknot the parts of your past that hold you back, you may trigger feelings of discomfort in others. Remember: how others behave towards your journey is not in your control, so don't try to control it! Throw the leaves in the air and let the wind carry them to where they're supposed to be. This is about you – and only you.

You have committed to yourself that it's time to unknot the learned behaviour of your past and the path of self-deprecation has come to an end. From now on, it's up to you to bring a sense of awareness in how you communicate about yourself and about others. You've come out of autopilot and you're getting into the driving seat. This is where you rise, where you carve out the existence you will choose to live! I'm excited for you! This. Is. It.

There aren't enough words in my vocabulary to express how proud I am of you. You have taken the time and energy to read this book, to digest these words and to begin to carve out your new ritualistic place of flow. You are creating a system that works for your day-to-day. You want more from life, and I want more for you. You are a powerful, incredible being and as your inner fire and confidence starts to bubble, peace and love will present itself to the onlooker, to the world ... and most importantly to the person you see looking back at you in the mirror every day. YOU. Vibe. High. Babes! You got this.

Acknowledgements

To my inner core energy radiators, what would I do with you?! My wonderful, incredible friends. Thank you for always being there to have deep, soulful, enriching conversations with. Thank you for being vulnerable with me, and for allowing me to do the same in return. Those moments we've shared have carved out more than we'll ever know. You have all helped me SO MUCH during this process, from sounding-out ideas, to inspiring me with your thoughts and feelings, and for endlessly lifting me up. You bloody legends.

There are so many people who, without them, this book wouldn't have been possible. Thank you to Kirsty and Holly and the wonderful team at Little, Brown who, when the world felt like it didn't want to hear my voice, told me to go for it and get writing! Thank you for holding my hand through this process. Just like Ariel says – a whole new world!

Thank you to my wonderful family for always being there during this journey, as I am here for you during yours. Finally, to my husband Dutch: *Ik hou van jou. Bedankt dat je mijn grootste supporter bent. Je bent de beste!* xx